Wow! 365 Easy Cookie Recipes

(Wow! 365 Easy Cookie Recipes - Volume 1)

Karen Hall

Content

365 Awesome Easy Cookie Recipes

***

1. 4 Ingredients Peanut Butter Cookies Recipe

Serving: 25 | Prep: | Cook: 8mins | Ready in:

Ingredients

- 1 cup granulated sugar
- 1 teaspoon baking soda (I use a little less-about 2/3 teaspoon)
- 1 large egg
- 1 cup 100% all natural peanut butter (creamy or crunchy)

Direction

- Preheat Oven 350.
- Mix sugar and baking soda together; stir in egg until well blended.
- Add peanut butter and stir until dough stiffens.
- I use a small (1 1/4" scoop) to form the 'balls'.
- You will need a fork and sugar for the cross-hatch marks.
- Hint: Use red sugar for creamy and green sugar for crunchy.
- Place 'balls' on baking sheet about 2" apart.
- Dip fork in sugar and very gently press cross hatch marks onto tops of 'balls'.
- Do not flatten out the 'balls' or the end result will be a burnt cookie!
- Place cookies in oven and set timer for 8 minutes.
- Check cookies; if the cookies are not firm to the touch, allow to bake for one-minute intervals (check after each minute) until firm.
- Some ovens are 'faster' and you can burn these cookies very quickly if not careful.
- Allow to cool on baking sheet for 4-5 minutes; removing to wire racks to finish cooling.
- Warning: these cookies will literally melt in your mouth. It is almost impossible to eat just one!

2. 5 Ingredient Peanut Butter And Banana Energy Bars

Serving: 9 | Prep: | Cook: 40mins | Ready in:

Ingredients

- 3 very ripe bananas
- 1 cup peanut butter
- 1/4 cup honey or maple syrup, for a vegan version
- 1 teaspoon cinnamon optional
- 1 teaspoon vanilla extract optional
- 2 cups old-fashioned oats
- 1 cup sliced almonds or other nut/seed combination

Direction

- Using a hand or standing mixer, mix the bananas, peanut butter (1 cup), honey (1/4 cup), cinnamon (1 teaspoon, optional), and vanilla extract (1 teaspoon, optional) until very smooth.
- Add oats (2 cups) and almonds (1 cup) and mix until combined.
- Turn out onto a parchment covered baking dish (about 9x9 inches). Press and flatten with a spatula until evenly distributed.
- Bake at 350 degrees for 30 minutes, or until golden brown on edges.
- Allow to cool completely before cutting bars.
- Store at room temperature for a week or freeze for up to 6 months in an airtight container or wrapped individually in plastic wrap.

- Notes
- Variations: Add chocolate chips, other spices like nutmeg, or other extracts like almond.
- For a nut-free version, use sunflower seed butter instead of peanut butter and use sunflower seeds and/or pumpkin seeds instead of almonds.
- If you're gluten-sensitive, make sure to buy gluten-free oats.
- If your peanut butter is salt-free, I recommend adding 1/4 teaspoon or so of kosher salt to the mix.
- Recommended Equipment
- 9x9 Baking Dish (or similar size)
- Hand mixer
- Nutrition
- Serving: 1bar | Calories: 278kcal | Carbohydrates: 28g | Protein: 9g | Fat: 16g | Saturated Fat: 3g | Sodium: 100mg | Potassium: 361mg | Fiber: 5g | Sugar: 12g | Vitamin A: 19IU | Vitamin C: 3mg | Calcium: 43mg | Iron: 1mg.

3. 5 Ingredient Nutella Cookies Recipe

Serving: 16 | Prep: | Cook: 10mins | Ready in:

Ingredients

- 1 cup flour
- 1 cup nutella chocolate hazelnut spread
- 1 egg
- 1/4 cup sugar
- 2 tbsp milk

Direction

- Preheat oven to 350oF.
- Combine all ingredients. Mix well. Form into walnut sized balls. Place on parchment paper lined cookie sheet. Pat down to 2-inch discs with ball of hand or bottom of a glass. Bake for 8-10 minutes until set & toothpick comes out clean.

4. A Very Chewy Molasses Cookie Without Eggs! Recipe

Serving: 0 | Prep: | Cook: 1hours | Ready in:

Ingredients

- 1 cup white sugar
- 1 cup shortening
- 1 cup dark molasses
- 2 teaspoons baking soda
- 1 teaspoon ground ginger
- 2 teaspoon ground cinnamon
- 4 cups all-purpose flour

Direction

- Preheat oven to 425 degrees F (220 degrees C). Lightly grease cookie sheets.
- In a large bowl, cream together the sugar and shortening until smooth. Stir in the molasses. Combine the baking soda, ginger, cinnamon and 3 3/4 cups of the flour; blend into the molasses mixture. Add more flour if necessary to make dough stiff enough to roll out. Use remaining flour to dust rolling surface. Roll dough out to 1/4 inch thickness and cut with cookie cutters. Or I just roll them into balls sprinkle with sugar and flatten with a glass!!
- Bake for 5 to 7 minutes in the preheated oven. Remove from baking sheets to cool on wire racks. DO NOT OVER BAKE!!!

5. Absolutely Amazing White Chocolate RAsberryCookies Recipe

Serving: 30 | Prep: | Cook: 7mins | Ready in:

Ingredients

- 11 ounces of white chocolate... either bakers bar or chips
- .5 cup of butter or margerine
- a cup of sugar
- a pinch of salt
- 2 eggs
- 2.75 or 23/4 cups of flour
- i dont really like shortening but you can put some in about 1/2 tsp.
- seedless rasberry jam

Direction

- 1. Grease baking sheet and set oven for 375
- 2. Chop 4 ounces of white chocolate... Set to the side
- 3. Put another 4 ounces into a pan and melt, stirring it a lot ... Cool
- 4. In separate bowl beat the butter with a mixer on high speed, then add the sugar, salt, and baking soda. Beat in melted white chocolate and eggs. Mix in flour. Stir in the remaining chopped white chocolate.
- 5. Bake for 7 to 9 minutes, cool and enjoy!!!
- Melt the jam and scoop a little on topo of each cookie
- (optional) drizzle melted white, milk, or dark chocolate over to make them look nicer =)

6. Accordian Treats Recipe

Serving: 12 | Prep: | Cook: 22mins | Ready in:

Ingredients

- 2 sheets heavy duty foil 1 yard each
- 3/4 cup butter softened
- 3/4 cup granulated sugar
- 1 teaspoon vanilla
- 2 eggs
- 1 cup all purpose flour
- 1/4 teaspoon salt
- 1/2 cup chopped walnuts

Direction

- Preheat oven to 325.
- Fold 1 sheet of foil in half lengthwise.
- Fold the double thickness foil crosswise into 1" pleats to make an accordion pleated pan.
- Place on cookie sheet then repeat with second sheet of foil.
- In large bowl beat margarine and sugar until light and fluffy.
- Add vanilla and eggs then beat well.
- Lightly spoon flour into measuring cup and level off.
- Add flour and salt then mix well.
- Stir in walnuts then drop rounded teaspoon of dough into each fold of foil.
- Bake at 325 for 22 minutes or until golden brown.
- Remove cookies from foil then cool completely.
- Turn foil over for second baking.

7. Aero Chocolate Biscuit Cake Recipe

Serving: 0 | Prep: | Cook: 25mins | Ready in:

Ingredients

- Aero chocolate (mint,orange or plain, your choice)
- digestive biscuits
- butter/oil
- greaseproof paper
- tin
- measure your ingredients to suit your needs.

Direction

- 1. Grease and line your tin with butter/oil and greaseproof paper
- 2. Break up your chocolate and place it a bowl. Then place your bowl over another bowl with boiling water in it. (You can also melt your chocolate in the microwave but it tends to burn more easily.)

3. While your chocolate is melting smash your biscuits into small chunks or crumbs.

4. Then fold in the biscuit into the fully melted chocolate, pour into tin and leave in the fridge to set overnight.

5. When set, slice into evenly cut squares. Place on a plate, serve up and enjoy.

8. Almond Bark Cookies Recipe

Serving: 25 | Prep: | Cook: 10mins | Ready in:

Ingredients

- 2 pounds almond bark
- 2 cups roasted peanuts
- 3 cups Rice Krispies cereal
- 1 cup chunky peanut butter
- 2 cups mini marshmellows

Direction

- Melt almond bark on top of stove or in the microwave.
- Stir in peanut butter until smooth.
- Add rest of ingredients and mix well.
- Drop by spoonful on wax paper.
- Makes 6 dozen.

9. Almond Biscotti Recipe

Serving: 0 | Prep: | Cook: 2hours | Ready in:

Ingredients

- 2 1/4 C Flour
- 1 C Sugar
- 1 t baking powder
- 1/2 t baking soda
- 1/2 t cinnamon
- 2 Eggs
- 2 Egg whites
- 1 T almond or vanilla extract
- 3/4 C Sliced almonds

Direction

- Preheat oven to 325.
- Combine dry ingredients in a medium mixing bowl.
- Whisk together eggs, egg whites, and extract in a separate mixing bowl.
- Add to dry ingredients, mixing just until moist.
- Add almonds and mix thoroughly. The dough will be sticky, but not so loose that it will not hold its shape. If it is too loose, gradually mix in small amounts of additional flour until the dough can hold its shape.
- On a floured surface, divide batter in half and pat each half into a log approximately 14 inches long.
- Bake for 30 minutes until firm.
- Cool on a wire rack.
- Reduce oven temperature to 300.
- Cut biscotti into 1⁄2-inch slices.
- Stand the slices upright (i.e. both cut sides exposed) on a cookie sheet.
- Bake for an additional 20 minutes.
- Let cool.
- Store in a loosely covered container.

10. Almond Butter Brickle Cookies Recipe

Serving: 24 | Prep: | Cook: 15mins | Ready in:

Ingredients

- 2 cups butter softened
- 2 cups granulated sugar
- 2 cups powdered sugar
- 2 cups vegetable oil
- 4 large eggs
- 2 teaspoons almond extract
- 9 cups all purpose flour
- 2 teaspoons baking soda

- 2 teaspoons cream of tartar
- 1-1/2 teaspoons salt
- 2 cups toasted almonds chopped
- 1 package butter brickle bits

Direction

- In mixing bowl cream butter and sugars then add oil, eggs and extract and mix well. Combine flour, soda, cream of tartar and salt and gradually add to creamed mixture.
- Stir in almonds and butter brickle bits then shape into balls and roll in granulated sugar.
- Flatten with fork and bake on ungreased cookie sheet at 350 for 14 minutes.

11. Almond Cookies Recipe

Serving: 24 | Prep: | Cook: 8mins | Ready in:

Ingredients

- 1/2 cup butter, softened
- 1/2 cup white sugar
- 1 egg
- 1 cup all-purpose flour
- 1 cup ground almonds (bake almonds on 350°F for 7 minutes and allow to cool before grinding)
- 1/2 t. almond extract or 2 t amaretto liqueur

Direction

- Preheat oven to 350°F
- In large bowl, cream together the butter and sugar. Beat in the egg, amaretto, and almonds. Gradually mix in the flour until well blended. Drop by teaspoonfuls 2 inches apart on ungreased cookie sheets.
- Bake 5 to 8 minutes in the preheated oven, or until cookies are lightly colored. Cookies do not spread - roll out

12. Almond Crunch Cookies Recipe

Serving: 24 | Prep: | Cook: 10mins | Ready in:

Ingredients

- 1 cup butter softened
- 3/4 cup firmly packed light brown sugar
- 1/2 cup granulated sugar
- 1 egg
- 1 teaspoon vanilla extract
- 2-1/4 cups all purpose flour
- 1/2 teaspoon baking soda
- 1/2 teaspoon cream of tartar
- 1-1/2 cups finely chopped almonds

Direction

- Beat butter at medium speed of an electric mixer then gradually add sugars mixing well.
- Add egg and vanilla then beat well.
- Combine flour, soda and cream of tartar then gradually add to creamed mixture.
- Mix well after each addition then stir in almonds.
- Drop cookie dough by rounded teaspoonfuls onto lightly greased cookie sheets.
- Bake at 350 for 10 minutes or until lightly browned.

13. Almond Lace Cookies By Juels Recipe

Serving: 8 | Prep: | Cook: 4mins | Ready in:

Ingredients

- • 1/2 cup chopped almonds (I measured out 3/4 cups of whole nuts, too much as you can see. When chopped the volume increased, probably no more than 1/4 + will create 1/2 cup)
- • 1/4 cup butter (1/2 of a cube, 4 tablespoons)
- • 1/3 cup all-purpose flour
- • 1/2 cup sugar

- • 2 tbsp. heavy cream
- • 1/2 tsp. vanilla OR almond extract (I used 1/4 tsp of each)
- • 3 oz semi-sweet chocolate chips (I used 1/3 cup)
- • 1 tbsp. shortening (I used 1 teaspoon)

Direction

- 1. Preheat the oven to 375F. Grease 2 baking sheets, or spray them with non-stick cooking spray.
- 2. Boil the chopped almonds for 2 min. in just enough water to cover them. Drain and use a food processor to chop finely.
- 3. Melt the butter in a saucepan over low heat. Remove from the heat and stir in the heavy cream and extract first so you get a through mix, then the flour and sugar. Last add the chopped nuts.
- 4. Drop teaspoonfuls 2 1/2 inches apart on the prepared cookie sheets. I found the correct amount is a level measuring teaspoon (see pic). The mixture slides right out of the spoon. As you can see in the pics I first used a regular spoon and then added the last amount in the bowl to each amount. Big mistake. This mixture really melts down. Yep the first batch turned into one big cookie. At about 2 minutes they start the big spread.
- 5. Bake until golden rims form, about 5 min. I found the time to be from 3 1/2 to 4 or as soon as the edges started to brown. I think the longer they cook, the crisper they will get, so if you want them chewier, very light brown edges, they turn quick, you cannot take your eyes off these when cooking.
- 6. I let them cool about 2-3 minutes on the cookie tray and then using a metal spatula I placed them on a piece of paper towel to absorb the butter that is on the bottom of the cookies, see pics.
- 7. Meanwhile, melt the chocolate chips with 1 tbsp. shortening in a microwave, about 1 min (use a microwave-safe bowl). Stir to make a smooth chocolate sauce. -- I melted the chips once the cookies where cooked. Drizzle the chocolate sauce over the lace cookies. -- I couldn't get the chocolate to drizzle so I loaded a spoon and just touched each cookie with the spoon to get the chocolate on the cookies, it worked for me.
- 8. It took a few hours for the chocolate to harden.

14. Almond Toffee Oatmeal Cookies Recipe

Serving: 24 | Prep: | Cook: 12mins | Ready in:

Ingredients

- Ingredients
- For the almond butter toffee
- 1/3 cup plus 1 tablespoon granulated sugar
- 1/4 cup unsalted butter
- 2 tablespoons water
- 1/8-1/4 teaspoon salt
- 1/3 cup flaked almonds
- For the cookies
- 1 cup all-purpose flour
- 1/2 teaspoon baking powder
- 1/2 teaspoon baking soda
- 1/4 teaspoon salt
- 1/2 cup butter
- 1/2 cup firmly-packed light brown sugar
- 2 tablespoons dark corn syrup, golden syrup, honey or maple syrup
- 1 egg
- 1 teaspoon pure vanilla extract
- 1 1/2 cups old-fashioned rolled oats
- 3/4 cup chocolate chips
- 1 batch almond butter toffee, crushed into bits

Direction

- To make the almond butter toffee: grease a half sheet pan (13"x18") or cookie sheet.
- Combine all ingredients, except the almonds, in a small, heavy bottomed saucepan. Over medium heat, stir until the butter is melted. Reduce the heat to medium-low and continue

to cook, stirring occasionally, until a candy thermometer reaches 300°F (150°C). This will take about 25-30 minutes. If you do not have a candy thermometer, carefully drip a small amount of the sugar mixture into a cup of cold water; if it has reached the right temperature it will collect into a hard ball.

- Meanwhile, in a skillet over medium-high heat, spread the almonds in a single layer. Toss the nuts occasionally to prevent scorching. Once they are light toasted brown and aromatic, remove from pan and set aside.
- Mix nuts into butter toffee mixture. Working quickly, spread the toffee over the prepared half sheet pan in a thin layer. It will not fill the entire pan. Set aside to cool completely.
- When cooled, break the toffee into irregular bits. I find it easiest to put pieces into a large, loosely sealed food storage bag and pounding the toffee into submission with the bottom of a skillet. You should end up with about 3/4 cup of nubby gravel.
- For the cookies: preheat the oven to 350°F (175°C).
- In a medium bowl, sift together the flour, baking powder, baking soda and salt. Set aside.
- In the bowl of a mixer fitted with the paddle attachment, or with a hand mixer, cream together the butter, brown sugar and corn syrup until light and fluffy. Scrape down the sides of the bowl as needed. Add the egg, beating well. Mix in vanilla.
- With mixer on low speed, add flour mixture and mix until just incorporated. Using a rubber spatula or wooden spoon, stir in the oatmeal, chocolate chips and crushed toffee.
- Drop 2 tablespoons of dough into mounds (I use a disher that is 1 1/2" across) onto parchment or Silpat lined cookie sheets. Space mounds about 2 inches apart. Bake until lightly golden around the edges, but not crisp, about 10-12 minutes.
- Cool on sheets for 5 minutes; transfer to a wire rack to cool completely.

15. Amaretto Cheesecake Cookies Recipe

Serving: 24 | Prep: | Cook: 25mins | Ready in:

Ingredients

- 1 cup all-purpose flour
- 1/3 cup brown sugar packed
- 6 tablespoons butter softened
- 8 ounces cream cheese softened
- 1/4 cup granulated sugar
- 1 egg
- 4 tablespoons Amaretto
- 1/2 teaspoon vanilla
- 4 tablespoons almonds chopped

Direction

- In large mixing bowl combine flour and brown sugar.
- Cut in butter until mixture forms fine crumbs.
- Reserve 1 cup crumb mixture for topping.
- Press remainder over bottom of ungreased square baking pan.
- Bake 15 minutes at 350.
- In mixer bowl thoroughly cream together cream cheese and granulated sugar.
- Add egg, amaretto and vanilla then beat well.
- Spread batter over partially baked crust.
- Combine almonds with reserved crumb mixture then sprinkle over batter.
- Bake 25 minutes then cool and cut into squares.

16. Amazing Cherry Chip Cookies Recipe

Serving: 36 | Prep: | Cook: 9mins | Ready in:

Ingredients

- 1 c butter or margarine, softened

14

- 1 c brown sugar
- 1/2 c white sugar
- 2 eggs
- 1/2 tsp almond extract
- 2 c flour (you may use 1 cup white flour & 1 cup whole wheat flour)
- 1 tsp baking soda
- 1/2 tsp salt
- 2 c uncooked quick oatmeal
- 1 c chocolate chips
- 1 c marachino cherries, chopped
- 1 c coconut

Direction

- 1 With mixer cream together softened butter and sugars and beat until fluffy.
- 2. Add eggs and almond extract. Beat well.
- 3. In a separate bowl, combine flour, soda, and salt.
- 4. Add dry ingredients to butter mixture and beat on low speed until well mixed.
- 5. By hand stir in remaining ingredients.
- 6. Drop by teaspoons onto ungreased cookie sheet.
- 7. Bake at 375 degrees for 8-10 minutes.
- 8. Cool 1 minute then remove to cooling rack.
- 9. Yields 36 cookies.

17. Amish Sugar Cookies Recipe

Serving: 0 | Prep: | Cook: 1hours | Ready in:

Ingredients

- • 1 cup butter, softened
- • 1 cup vegetable oil
- • 1 cup sugar
- • 1 cup confectioners' sugar
- • 2 eggs
- • 1 teaspoon vanilla extract
- • 1 teaspoon almond extract
- • 4-1/2 cups all-purpose flour
- • 1 teaspoon baking soda
- • 1 teaspoon cream of tartar

Direction

- Preheat oven to 375° F.
- In large mixer bowl, beat the butter, oil and sugars thoroughly.
- Beat in eggs, vanilla and almond extract until well blended.
- Combine the flour, baking soda and cream of tartar; gradually add to butter and sugar mixture.
- Drop by tablespoonfuls onto ungreased baking sheets. Bake for 8-10 minutes, or until lightly browned around the edges. Remove to wire racks to cool.
- These would be great chilled and rolled in cinnamon and sugar like a snicker doodle, but I think I am also going to try adding fiori di sicilia and/or orange extract the next time I make them!

18. Angelic Cookies Recipe

Serving: 12 | Prep: | Cook: 8mins | Ready in:

Ingredients

- 1 recipe butter cookie Dough (recipe follows)
- 1 egg, lightly beaten
- small pretzels, white frosting, toasted coconut, edible glitter dust and assorted small decors

Direction

- Preparation:
- Prepare and chill Butter Cookie Dough as directed.
- Preheat oven to 350°F.
- Grease cookie sheets.
- Roll dough on floured surface to 1/4-inch thickness.
- Cut out 12 (4-inch) triangles.
- Reroll scraps to 1/4-inch thickness.
- Cut out 12 (1-1/2-inch) circles.
- Place triangles on prepared cookie sheets.
- Brush with beaten egg.

- Attach circle, pressing gently.
- Bake 8 to 10 minutes or just until edges begin to brown.
- Remove to wire racks; cool completely.
- Attach pretzels to back of each cookie for wings using frosting as "glue." Let stand 30 minutes or until frosting is set.
- Pipe frosting around hairline of each angel; sprinkle with coconut and glitter dust.
- Decorate cookies with frosting, coconut, glitter dust and decors to resemble angels as desired.
- Let cookies stand 1 hour or until frosting is set.
- You can make royal icing to use on these cookies as well.
- Butter Cookie Dough
- Ingredients:
- 3/4 cup (1-1/2 sticks) butter, softened
- 1/4 cup granulated sugar
- 1/4 cup packed light brown sugar
- 1 egg yolk
- 1-3/4 cups all-purpose flour
- 3/4 teaspoon baking powder
- 1/8 teaspoon salt
- Preparation:
- 1. Combine butter, granulated sugar, brown sugar and egg yolk in medium bowl. Add flour, baking powder and salt; mix well.
- 2. Cover; refrigerate about 4 hours or until firm.

19. Anise Biscotti Recipe

Serving: 24 | Prep: | Cook: 25mins | Ready in:

Ingredients

- 1 cup granulated sugar
- 1/2 cup sweet butter melted
- 3 tablespoons Anisette
- 2 teaspoons anise seeds
- 1 teaspoon vanilla
- 1 cup unsalted almonds chopped
- 3 eggs
- 2-1/2 cups flour

- 1/2 tablespoon baking powder
- 1/4 teaspoon salt

Direction

- Preheat oven to 350.
- Mix sugar with butter, anisette, anise seeds, vanilla, nuts and eggs then mix well.
- Stir in flour, baking powder and salt then form into a long loaf and place on cookie sheet.
- Bake 30 minutes or until firm and softly cake like then remove from oven and cool slightly.
- When cool enough to handle slice into 1/2" diagonal slices and return to cookie sheet.
- Bake 20 minutes long turning once until both sides are brown flecked and toasted.
- Cool thoroughly and store in airtight jar.

20. Anisette Toast Recipe

Serving: 24 | Prep: | Cook: 45mins | Ready in:

Ingredients

- 2 1/2 cups all-purpose flour
- 2 teaspoons baking powder
- 1/4 teaspoon baking soda
- 1/4 teaspoon salt
- 1/4 cup softened butter
- 1 cup white sugar
- 3 eggs
- 4 teaspoons anise extract

Direction

- 1. Preheat an oven to 350 degrees F (175 degrees C). Whisk together the flour, baking powder, baking soda, and salt in a bowl; set aside. Line 2 baking sheets with parchment paper.
- 2. Beat the butter and sugar with an electric mixer in a large bowl until fluffy. Beat in one egg until completely incorporated, then another. Beat in the last egg along with the anise extract. Mix in the flour until just

incorporated. Divide the dough onto the prepared baking sheets. Form each portion into a 12-inch long log, 1/2-inch thick.

- 3. Bake in the preheated oven until golden and firm to the touch, 20 to 25 minutes. Remove from the oven, and allow to cool 5 minutes. Cut into 3/4-inch thick slices using a serrated knife, and place cut-side-down onto the baking sheets. Return to the oven, and bake 5 to 10 minutes until the bottoms turn golden brown. Turn the cookies over, and continue baking until golden brown on the other side, 5 to 10 minutes more. Cool completely on a wire rack before serving.

21. Apple Butter Peanut Butter Cookies Recipe

Serving: 12 | Prep: | Cook: 12mins | Ready in:

Ingredients

- 1 cup apple butter
- 1/2 cup natural style chunky peanut butter
- 1 teaspoon vanilla
- 3/4 cup powdered milk
- 3/4 cup whole wheat flour
- 1/2 teaspoon salt
- 1/2 teaspoon ground cinnamon
- 1/2 cup raisins

Direction

- Prepare cookie sheet with oil then preheat oven to 350.
- In a large bowl beat apple butter, peanut butter and vanilla then set aside.
- Stir together in a medium bowl powdered milk, flour, salt, cinnamon and raisins.
- Add dry ingredients to apple butter mixture and mix well.
- Drop by teaspoon onto prepared cookie sheet.
- Flatten with fork dipped in ice water making a crisscross pattern on top.

- Bake at 350 for 10 minutes then cool and refrigerate until well chilled then serve cold.

22. Apple Buttery Sweet Crumbly Elegant Light Recipe

Serving: 16 | Prep: | Cook: 25mins | Ready in:

Ingredients

- 1 cup brown sugar firmly packed
- 1-1/2 cups flour
- 3/4 cup butter
- 1-1/2 cups oatmeal
- 1/2 teaspoon baking soda
- 1 teaspoon vanilla extract
- 1/2 teaspoon salt
- 2 cups apple butter
- powdered sugar

Direction

- Mix all ingredients except apple butter until crumbly.
- Spread 1/2 of the mixture into a greased rectangular pan.
- Spread apple butter over crumbly mixture then cover with remaining crumbs.
- Bake at 350 for 25 minutes.
- Allow to cool for a few minutes then sprinkle with powdered sugar.

23. Applesauce Bars Recipe

Serving: 36 | Prep: | Cook: 27mins | Ready in:

Ingredients

- 1/2 cup shortening
- 1 cup packed light brown sugar
- 1 egg
- 1-3/4 cups all-purpose flour

- 1/2 teaspoon baking soda
- 1/2 teaspoon salt
- 1/2 teaspoon ground cinnamon
- 1/4 teaspoon ground nutmeg
- 1/4 teaspoon ground cloves
- 1 cup thick applesauce
- 1/4 cup water
- 1-2/3 cups (10-oz. pkg.) REESE'S peanut butter chips or HERSHEY'S cinnamon Chips
- 1/2 cup golden raisins(optional)
- lemon FROSTING(recipe follows)

Direction

- Directions:
- 1. Heat oven to 400°F. Grease 13x9x2-inch baking pan.
- 2. Beat shortening, brown sugar and egg until light and fluffy in large bowl. Stir together flour, baking soda, salt, cinnamon, nutmeg and cloves; add to shortening mixture, beating until well blended. Add applesauce and water; beat until well blended. Stir in peanut butter chips and raisins, if desired. Spread batter in prepared pan.
- 3. Bake 25 to 30 minutes or until wooden pick inserted in centre comes out clean. Cool slightly in pan on wire rack. Frost with LEMON FROSTING.* Cut into bars. About 36 bars.
- LEMON FROSTING
- 2-1/2 tablespoons butter or margarine, softened
- 1-1/2 cups powdered sugar
- 4 to 4-1/2 teaspoons lemon juice
- 1 teaspoon freshly grated lemon peel
- Beat butter and powdered sugar in small bowl until well blended. Gradually add lemon juice and peel; beat until of spreading consistency. About 3/4 cup frosting.
- * Recipe may be doubled for a thicker frosting. Original recipe amount is more like a glaze.

24. Applesauce Spice Cookies Dated 1966 Recipe

Serving: 24 | Prep: | Cook: 15mins |Ready in:

Ingredients

- 1 cup raisins
- 1 cup canned applesauce
- 1 cup brown sugar
- 1/2 cup shortening
- 1 egg
- 2 cups all-purpose flour
- 1/2 teaspoon salt
- 1 teaspoon baking soda
- 1 teaspoon cinnamon
- 1 teaspoon nutmeg
- 1/4 teaspoon ground cloves
- 1 cup chopped nuts

Direction

- Preheat oven to 350.
- Mix raisins with applesauce then set aside.
- Beat sugar and shortening then add egg and beat until fluffy.
- Stir in applesauce raisin mixture.
- Sift dry ingredients together then add to wet mixture and stir in nuts.
- Drop by teaspoonfuls on cookie sheet. Then bake 15 minutes.

25. Apricot Buttons Recipe

Serving: 24 | Prep: | Cook: 20mins |Ready in:

Ingredients

- 1/2 cup dried apricots
- 2/3 cup sugar
- 1/2 cup butter
- 1 egg, separated
- 1/4 tsp. pure vanilla extract or pure almond extract

- Note: I prefer almond extract with these cookies
- 1/2 tsp. salt
- 1/4 tsp. bkg. soda (the baking soda can be omitted)
- 1 cup flour
- 3/4 cup finely chopped pecans

Direction

- Combine apricots and 1/3 cup of the sugar; cook until thickened. Cool and set aside.
- Cream butter and remaining sugar until light and fluffy.
- Beat in egg yolk and vanilla.
- Sift salt, baking soda and flour together and add to creamed mixture.
- Chill dough slightly.
- Form into balls.
- Slightly beat egg white.
- Dip cookies in egg white, then in pecans.
- Place on greased cookie sheet. With your thumb, make indentation in center of each.
- Bake at 350 degrees F for 20 minutes.
- While still warm, fill centers with apricot mixture.
- Apricot preserves may be substituted for dried apricots!
- Note: If your dough appears too thin, just add more flour.

26. Apricot Cream Cheese Bars Recipe

Serving: 12 | Prep: | Cook: 45mins | Ready in:

Ingredients

- 1 package French vanilla cake mix
- 1/3 cup butter melted
- 1 egg
- 12 ounce jar apricot preserves
- 8 ounce package cream cheese softened
- 1/4 cup granulated sugar

- 1/2 teaspoon vanilla
- 1 egg

Direction

- Preheat oven to 350 then grease a rectangular pan.
- In a large bowl combine cake mix, butter and egg then mix with fork until just crumbly.
- Gently spoon 1-1/2 cups into measuring cup and set aside for topping.
- Press remainder of crumb mixture into bottom of pan and bake 10 minutes.
- Spread preserves over baked crust.
- In a small bowl combine cream cheese, sugar, vanilla and egg then beat until smooth.
- Spread over preserves then sprinkle reserved topping mix over cream cheese mixture.
- Bake 30 minutes then chill and cut into squares.
- Store leftovers in refrigerator.

27. Apricot Oatmeal Bars Recipe

Serving: 28 | Prep: | Cook: 25mins | Ready in:

Ingredients

- 1 C all purpose flour
- 1 c quick cooking oats
- 1 tsp salt
- 1/2 tsp cinnamon
- 1/4 tsp ground cloves
- 1 tsp baking soda
- 6 TBLS butter
- 6 TBLS canola oil
- 3/4 c white sugar - I use half sugar & half splenda
- 1/2 c brown sugar
- 2 eggs
- 1 tsp vanilla
- 1/2 c dried apricots, diced - any dried fruit will work here

Direction

- Preheat oven to 375. Spray a 9x13 with non-stick spray - pam.
- Combine first 5 ingredients in one bowl, set aside.
- Combine butter through vanilla in another bowl and mix with electric mixer till smooth and fluffy.
- Add dry ingredients to the wet and mix just till incorporated. Add dried fruit.
- Spread mixture evenly into prepared pan, bake for 20-25 min. Cool completely before cutting into bars.

28. Apricot Walnuts Bars Recipe

Serving: 24 | Prep: | Cook: 25mins | Ready in:

Ingredients

- 1 cup butter
- 1/2 cup granulated sugar
- 2 cups flour
- Filling:
- 1-1/3 cup dried apricots
- 2/3 cup all purpose flour
- 1 teaspoon baking powder
- 1/2 teaspoon salt
- 2 cup brown sugar packed
- 4 large eggs
- 1 cup chopped walnuts
- 1 teaspoon vanilla extract
- 1/2 cup powdered sugar

Direction

- Preheat oven to 350.
- Cream butter and sugar then stir in flour until crumbly then pack into rectangular baking pan.
- Bake 25 minutes or until lightly browned.
- Cook apricots in small amount of water until softened.
- Drain and process until pureed in food processor.

- Beat brown sugar and eggs together until well blended then add dry and mix until blended.
- Add vanilla, apricots and nuts then mix until blended and spread over baked layer.
- Bake 25 minutes until golden then cool and sprinkle with powdered sugar then cut into pieces.

29. Armenian Almond Cookies Recipe

Serving: 24 | Prep: | Cook: 20mins | Ready in:

Ingredients

- 1 cup butter
- 1/2 cup sugar
- 2 cups flour
- 1/2 tsp salt
- 1 Tbs vanilla
- 1 tsp almond extract
- 1/2 cup chopped almonds or walnuts
- 24 blanched almonds

Direction

- Cream butter and sugar.
- Blend in flavorings and chopped nuts
- Mix together dry ingredients.
- Mix into creamed mixture with electric mixer until well blended.
- Shape into small balls the size of walnuts
- Place on an ungreased baking sheet and flatten with a fork.
- Place an almond in center of cookie
- Bake in a slow oven, 325F about 20 minutes or done

30. Austrian Chocolate Walnut Bars Recipe

Serving: 40 | Prep: | Cook: 40mins | Ready in:

Ingredients

- 1 cup butter, softened
- 1/2 cup packed brown sugar
- 2-1/2 cups all-purpose flour
- 2/3 cup apricot preserves
- 4 eggs
- 1-1/2 cups packed brown sugar
- 1/4 cup unsweetened Dutch-process cocoa powder
- 2 teaspoons vanilla
- 1 teaspoon salt
- 3 cups walnuts, toasted and finely ground*
- 8 ounces bittersweet chocolate, chopped
- 3 tablespoons butter
- 1 tablespoon light-color corn syrup
- 1 tablespoon rum
- About 40 walnut halves, toasted (optional)

Direction

- 1. Preheat oven to 375 degrees F. Grease a 13x9x2-inch baking pan; set aside. In a large bowl, beat the 1 cup butter with an electric mixer on medium to high speed for 30 seconds. Add the 1/2 cup brown sugar. Beat until combined, scraping side of bowl occasionally. Gradually add flour, beating on low speed just until combined (mixture will look slightly dry). Press mixture into prepared pan. Bake in the preheated oven for 10 minutes. Carefully spread preserves over hot crust.
- 2. In another large bowl, beat eggs on medium-high speed for 3 minutes. Add the 1-1/2 cups brown sugar, the cocoa powder, vanilla, and salt. Beat on low speed for 3 minutes. Gradually add the finely ground walnuts, beating just until combined.
- 3. Carefully spread chocolate mixture evenly over preserves. Bake about 30 minutes or until set. Cool completely in pan on a wire rack.
- 4. For icing: In a medium heavy saucepan, combine bittersweet chocolate and the 3 tablespoons butter. Cook and stir over low heat until melted. Stir in corn syrup and rum. Spread icing over cooled uncut cookies. If

desired, top with the walnut halves. Let stand for 1 to 2 hours or until chocolate is set. Using a sharp knife, loosen edges of cookies from sides of pan. Cut into bars. Makes about 40 bars.

- 5. *Test Kitchen Tip: To prevent overgrinding the nuts and turning them into a paste, grind about one-third at a time.
- 6. To Store: Place bars in a single layer in an airtight container; cover. Store at room temperature for up to 3 days or freeze for up to 3 months.

31. Awesome Almond Shortbread Recipe

Serving: 20 | Prep: | Cook: 20mins | Ready in:

Ingredients

- 3/4 lb. butter at room temp.
- 1c. sugar
- 5 teaspoons of almond extract
- 1 teaspoon of vanilla extract
- 31/2c. All Purpose flour
- 1/2 teaspoon salt
- 11/2c. sliced almonds

Direction

- Preheat oven to 350
- Beat butter and sugar till combined
- Add extracts
- In another bowl sift flour and salt
- Add flour mixture to sugar mixture
- Add almonds
- Mix just till it comes together
- Shape into a disk and chill 30 min
- Roll 1/2in. thick and cut in desired shapes
- Bake on ungreased cookie sheet for 20-25 min.

32. BAVARIAN CLOUD CAKE WITH TEA LACED WHIPPED CREAM Recipe

Serving: 12 | Prep: | Cook: 28mins | Ready in:

Ingredients

- 1 1/3 cups boiling water
- 2 Lipton Bavarian Wild Berry Pyramid tea bags
- 1 box of your favorite chocolate cake mix
- 1/3 cup vegetable oil
- 3 eggs

Direction

- Pour boiling water over tea bags; cover and brew about 5 minutes.
- Remove tea bags (squeeze); and cool.
- Preheat oven to 350.
- Grease and lightly flour two 9-inch round cake pans; set aside.
- In a large bowl, with electric mixer on low speed, beat cake mix, brewed tea, oil and eggs 30 seconds or just until moistened.
- Continue to beat on medium speed (scraping the sides occasionally) for 2 minutes.
- Pour batter into prepared pans.
- Bake 28 minutes or until toothpick inserted in center comes out clean.
- Cool on wire rack for 10 minutes.
- Serve with tea-laced whipped cream.
- Tea-Laced Whipped Cream:
- Steep 3 Lipton Bavarian Wild Berry Pyramid Tea Bags in 1/4 cup boiling water for 5 minutes; remove tea bags and squeeze.
- Stir in 1/4 cup sugar until dissolved and chill.
- Beat cooled tea with 1 pint whipping cream until soft peaks form.

33. BEST Granola Bars Ever Recipe

Serving: 14 | Prep: | Cook: 5mins | Ready in:

Ingredients

- GRAINS:
- 1 cup rice puffs
- 1 cup rolled oats
- 1 cup rolled wheat
- 1/2 chopped almonds
- 1/2 sunflower seeds
- 1/2 cup flax seeds
- 1/2 cup dried cranberries
- GLAZE:
- 2/3 cup light brown sugar
- 1/3 cup + 1 TBS honey
- 1/4 cup butter (half a stick)
- 1 tsp vanilla

Direction

- Toast any raw grains in the oven for about 5 min. at 400 degrees, mixing half-way thru.
- Line 13x9 inch pan with foil to spread granola in.
- Mix all dry ingredients in very large bowl, or stock pot (I like to use my 8 qt. pot).
- Heat all glaze ingredients in heavy sauce pan on stove top at medium heat.
- Bring to boil, reduce heat stirring constantly, and simmer 2 minutes.
- Pour glaze over dry ingredients, mix well.
- Spread in foil lined pan, smooth flat with back of spoon.
- Smooth a LOT, as you want the grains to be packed together so the bars don't fall apart!
- Let sit for 2 hours.
- Remove granola in foil and place on counter, using a large knife, cut into bars.
- I like to individually wrap the bars in sandwich bags, because I found out the hard way, that they stick together!

34. Baby Ruth Bars Recipe

Serving: 36 | Prep: | Cook: 20mins | Ready in:

Ingredients

- 2 1/4 cups all-purpose flour
- 1 teaspoon baking soda
- 1/2 teaspoon salt
- 3/4 cup packed brown sugar
- 3/4 cup granulated sugar
- 1/2 cup butter OR margarine, softened
- 1/2 cup creamy OR chunky peanut butter
- 2 large eggs
- 1 teaspoon vanilla extract
- 6 (2.1-ounce each) Baby Ruth Candy Bars, coarsely chopped

Direction

- Preheat oven to 375° F.
- Grease 15 x 10-inch jelly roll pan.
- Combine flour, baking soda and salt in small bowl.
- Beat brown sugar, granulated sugar, butter and peanut butter in large mixer bowl until creamy.
- Beat in eggs and vanilla extract.
- Gradually beat in flour mixture.
- Spread dough evenly into prepared pan.
- Sprinkle with Baby Ruth; press in lightly.
- Bake for 18 to 20 minutes or until golden brown.
- Cool completely in pan on wire rack.
- Cut into bars.

35. Banana Bars Recipe

Serving: 36 | Prep: | Cook: 25mins | Ready in:

Ingredients

- 1/4 cup shortening
- 1 cup sugar
- 2 eggs
- 1 cup mashed bananas (2 to 3)
- 1 tsp. vanilla
- 2 cups all-purpose flour
- 2 tsp. baking powder
- 1/2 tsp. salt

Direction

- Heat oven to 350 degrees.
- Grease a jelly roll pan.
- Mix shortening, sugar, eggs, bananas, and vanilla thoroughly.
- Measure flour and blend the dry ingredients.
- Stir dry mixture into banana mixture.
- Spread in prepared pan.
- Bake 20 to 25 minutes or until golden brown.

36. Banana Split Cheesecake Squares Recipe

Serving: 1 | Prep: | Cook: 30mins | Ready in:

Ingredients

- Crust:
- 2 cups graham cracker crumbs
- 1/3 cup melted butter
- ¼ cup sugar
- Filling:
- 3 pkgs (8 oz. each) cream cheese
- ¾ cup sugar
- 1 tsp. vanilla
- 3 eggs
- ½ cup mashed banana
- Topping:
- 1 cup sliced strawberries
- 1 banana, sliced, tossed with 1 tsp. lemon juice
- 1 can (8 oz.) pineapple chunks, drained

Direction

- Crust:
- Mix crumbs, butter and sugar. Press onto bottom of 13x9x2 pan.
- Filling:
- Mix cream cheese, sugar and vanilla with electric mixer on medium speed until well blended. Add eggs; mix until blended. Stir in mashed banana. Pour into crust.
- Bake at 350 for 30 minutes or until center is almost set. Cool.

- Refrigerate 3 hours or overnight.
- Topping:
- Top with strawberries, sliced banana and pineapple. Drizzle with melted chocolate. Cut into squares.

37. Ben And Jerrys Giant Chocolate Chip Cookies Recipe

Serving: 1 | Prep: | Cook: 13mins | Ready in:

Ingredients

- 1/2 cup butter, room temperature
- 1/4 cup Granulated sugar
- 1/3 cup brown sugar
- 1 Large egg
- 1/2 teas vanilla extract
- 1 cup (+ 2 teas) All Purpose flour
- 1/2 teas salt
- 1/2 teas baking soda
- 1 cup semisweet chocolate chips
- 1/2 cup Coarsely Chopped walnuts

Direction

- Preheat the oven to 350F.
- Beat the butter and both sugars in a large mixing bowl until light and fluffy. Add the egg and vanilla extract and mix well.
- Mix the flour, salt, and baking soda in another bowl. Add the dry ingredients to the batter and mix until well blended. Stir in the chocolate chips and walnuts.
- Drop the dough by small scoops 2 to 3 inches apart on an ungreased cookie sheet. Flatten each scoop with the back of a spoon to about 3 inches in diameter.
- Bake until the centers are still slightly soft to the touch, 11 to 14 minutes. Let cool on the cookie sheet for 5 minutes, then transfer to racks to cool completely.
- Makes 12 to 15 cookies.

38. Best Chocolate Chip Cookies In The World Recipe

Serving: 1 | Prep: | Cook: 9mins | Ready in:

Ingredients

- 1 cup shortening
- 1/2 cup granulated sugar
- 1 cup packed brown sugar
- 2 eggs
- 2 teaspoons vanilla
- 2 cups all-purpose flour
- 1 teaspoon baking soda
- 1/2 teaspoon salt
- 1 1/2 - 2 cups chocolate chips

Direction

- Preheat oven to 375 degrees.
- Cream together the shortening and both sugars. Then add eggs, vanilla, flour, baking soda and salt. Once the shortening, sugar, eggs, vanilla, flour, baking soda and salt mixture is all creamed together, add the chocolate chips. Mix together, well.
- Drop cookie dough by teaspoonfuls onto ungreased cookie sheets and bake for about 9-12 minutes or until golden brown.

39. Best Ever Lemon Bars Recipe

Serving: 16 | Prep: | Cook: 33mins | Ready in:

Ingredients

- Crust Ingredients:
- 1 cup all-purpose flour
- 1/2 cup butter, softened
- 1/4 cup sugar
- Filling Ingredients:
- 3/4 cup sugar
- 2 eggs

- 2 tablespoons all-purpose flour
- 3 tablespoons lemon juice
- 1 teaspoon freshly grated lemon zest
- 1/4 teaspoon baking powder
- Topping Ingredients:
- powdered sugar

Direction

- Heat oven to 350°F. Combine all crust ingredients in small bowl. Beat at low speed, scraping bowl often, until mixture resembles coarse crumbs. Press onto bottom of ungreased 8-inch square baking pan. Bake for 15 to 20 minutes or until edges are lightly browned.
- Meanwhile, combine all filling ingredients except powdered sugar in small bowl. Beat at low speed, scraping bowl often, until well mixed. Pour filling over hot, partially baked crust. Continue baking for 18 to 20 minutes or until filling is set.
- Sprinkle with powdered sugar while still warm and again when cool. Cut into bars.

40. Best Ever Snowball Cookies Recipe

Serving: 8 | Prep: | Cook: 15mins | Ready in:

Ingredients

- 2 sticks (1 cup) cold unsalted butter, cut in small pieces
- 1/4 cup powdered sugar & 1 cup for rolling cookies in
- 2 tsp vanilla extract
- 2 cups all-purpose flour

Direction

- Heat oven to 350 degrees F
- In a large mixing bowl add butter, 1/4 powdered sugar and the vanilla. Process, scraping bowl often to blend.

- Add flour, about 1/2 cup at a time; process until combined.
- With lightly floured hands, roll dough into 1-inch balls.
- Place 1 inch apart on un-greased cookie sheets.
- Bake about 15 minutes until bottoms are light brown.
- Cool on wax paper on a wire rack for 15 minutes.
- Gently (cookies are fragile) roll warm cookies in 1 cup powdered sugar.
- Cool, then roll in sugar again.
- Refrigerate tightly covered with wax paper between layers up to 1 week.

41. Best Tasting Soft Chocolate Chip Cookies Recipe

Serving: 48 | Prep: | Cook: 12mins | Ready in:

Ingredients

- 1 cup butter, softened
- 3/4 cup packed brown sugar
- 1/4 cup white sugar
- 1 (3.5 oz) package instant vanilla pudding - secret ingredient
- 2 eggs
- 1-1/2 tsp. vanilla extract
- 2-1/4 cups all-purpose flour
- 1 tsp. baking soda
- 1/2 tsp. salt
- 2 cups semisweet chocolate chips or butterscotch chips
- *If I'm using instant vanilla pudding, I add butterscotch chips but if I use Instant chocolate pudding then I add the semi-sweet chocolate chips.
- My Note: If you really want a chocolate, chocolate chip cookie. Instead of using instant vanilla pudding use Instant chocolate pudding. Ohhhhhhhhhh yummmmmmmmm!!!

Direction

- Preheat oven to 375 degrees F (190 deg C).
- In a mixing bowl, cream butter and sugars.
- Add pudding mix, eggs, and vanilla.
- Combine flour, salt and baking soda.
- Add to creamed mixture and mix well.
- Fold in chocolate chips.
- Drop by rounded teaspoonful onto ungreased baking sheets.
- Bake for 10-12 minutes or until lightly browned at edges of cookie. These cookies do not spread out like your typical Toll house cookie.

42. Biscotti Recipe

Serving: 24 | Prep: | Cook: 60mins | Ready in:

Ingredients

- 2 cups all-purpose flour
- 2/3 cup sugar
- 1 tsp baking soda
- 1/2 tsp salt
- 1 tsp vanilla extract
- 2 tsp Creme de Cacao (optional)
- 3 large eggs, beaten
- 1/4 tsp cinnamon

Direction

- In a bowl, mix flour, sugar, soda, cinnamon, and salt
- Add eggs and vanilla, stirring until blended
- Turn dough out onto a floured surface
- Knead 8 - 10 times
- Form dough into a log about 2x16 inches
- Put log on a non-stick baking sheet (or one coated with non-stick spray)
- Bake in a preheated 350 degree oven for 30 minutes
- Remove and cool for 10 minutes
- Place the loaf on a cutting board and with a serrated knife cut 1/2 inch wide slices on the diagonal
- Place slices on their sides on the baking sheet

- Reduce oven to 325 degrees
- Bake biscotti for 10 more minutes
- Flip all slices and bake for another 10 to 12 minutes.
- Remove from oven and place on a rack to cool.

43. Black Forest Cookies Recipe

Serving: 30 | Prep: | Cook: 13mins | Ready in:

Ingredients

- 1 11.5-ounce package milk chocolate morsels, divided
- 1/2 cup brown sugar
- 1/4 cup butter, softened
- 2 eggs
- 1 teaspoon vanilla extract
- 3/4 cup flour
- 1/4 teaspoon baking powder
- 1 6-ounce package craisins,Cherry Flavor
- Sweetened dried cranberries
- 1 cup pecans or walnuts, coarsely chopped

Direction

- Preheat oven to 350° F.
- Pour 3/4 cup morsels into an uncovered large microwave-safe bowl. Set remaining morsels aside. Microwave morsels for 2 minutes on high. Stir until chocolate is smooth.
- Stir in brown sugar, butter, eggs and vanilla. Add flour and baking powder, mixing until thoroughly combined. Stir in remaining morsels, cherry flavour sweetened dried cranberries and pecans.
- Drop by tablespoonfuls onto a greased cookie sheet. Bake for 12 minutes or until cookies are puffed and set to the touch. For a firmer cookie bake for 14 minutes. Cool on cookie sheet for 2 minutes. Transfer to a wire rack and cool completely. Makes about 2 1/2 dozen cookies

44. Black Magic Cookies With Blackstrap Icing Recipe

Serving: 24 | Prep: | Cook: 30mins | Ready in:

Ingredients

- 1 cup raisins
- 1/4 cup dark rum
- 3 cups flour
- 1/4 cup unsweetened cocoa
- 2 tablespoons baking powder
- 1/2 teaspoon ground allspice
- 1/2 teaspoon ground cinnamon
- 1/8 teaspoon salt
- 8 ounces semisweet chocolate cut into 1/4" pieces
- 1/2 pound unsalted butter cut into 1 ounce pieces
- 1 cup firmly packed brown sugar
- 3 large eggs
- 1 teaspoon vanilla
- Icing:
- 6 ounces semisweet chocolate cut into 1/4" pieces
- 3/4 cup heavy cream
- 1/4 pound unsalted butter cut into 1 ounce pieces
- 2 tablespoons blackstrap molasses

Direction

- Combine raisins and rum in a plastic container with tight fitting lid.
- Steep at room temp for 6 hours or overnight.
- Preheat oven to 350.
- In a sifter combine flour, cocoa, baking powder, allspice, cinnamon and salt.
- Sift onto wax paper and set aside until needed.
- Heat 1" water in bottom half of a double boiler over medium heat.
- With heat on place chocolate in top half.
- Use a rubber spatula to stir chocolate until completely melted and smooth.
- Transfer melted chocolate to a 1-quart bowl and set aside until needed.
- Combine butter and brown sugar in bowl of an electric mixer fitted with a paddle.
- Beat on medium speed for 4 minutes using rubber spatula to scrape down sides of bowl.
- Continue to beat on medium 4 more minutes until fairly smooth.
- Scrape down bowl then beat on high for 2 minutes until smooth.
- Add eggs one at a time beating on medium 1 minute and scraping down bowl after each addition.
- Add vanilla and beat on high 1 minute then scrape down bowl.
- Add melted chocolate and beat on medium 30 seconds until incorporated.
- Add rum infused raisins and mix on low for 30 seconds until combined scraping down bowl.
- Operate mixer on low while gradually adding dry ingredients.
- When all dry ingredients have been incorporated remove bowl from mixer.
- Use a rubber spatula to finish mixing the dough until thoroughly combined.
- Using heaping tablespoon dough for each cookie portion 12 cookies evenly spaced onto 4 sheets.
- Place sheets on top and center racks of preheated oven and bake 10 minutes rotating sheets.
- Remove cookies from oven and cool to room temperature on baking sheets about 30 minutes.
- To make icing place chocolate in a 3-quart bowl.
- Heat heavy cream, butter and molasses in a 1-1/2-quart saucepan over medium heat.
- Stir to dissolve molasses then bring to a boil.
- Pour boiling mixture over chocolate and set aside 5 minutes then stir until smooth.
- Keep icing at room temperature for 1 hour before using.
- Ice the cookies by spooning about 1 tablespoon atop each one.

45. Blitzen Bars Recipe

Serving: 24 | Prep: | Cook: 20mins | Ready in:

Ingredients

- 16 oz. pkg caramels
- 1 chocolate cake mix
- 1 cup nuts, chopped
- 2/3 cup evaporated milk
- 2/3 cup butter, melted
- 1 cup chocolate chips

Direction

- Preheat oven to 350 F.
- Combine caramels in 1/3 cup evaporated milk in saucepan, heat and stir until melted. Combine cake mix, butter and 1/3 cup evaporated milk and mix well. Press 1/2 of this dough into a 9" x 13" pan. Bake 5 minutes at 350 F. Sprinkle nuts and chocolate chips on baked dough. Cover with caramel mixture. Spread remaining half of dough over caramel. Spread with fingers (does not spread well). Bake 15 to 20 minutes at 350 F.

46. Blonde Spice Cookies Recipe

Serving: 5 | Prep: | Cook: 14mins | Ready in:

Ingredients

- 1 Cup butter (softened)
- 1/2 Cup Granulated sugar
- 1/2 Cup brown sugar
- 1   egg
- 2-1/2 Cups flour
- 3/4 Tsp baking soda
- 1/2 Tsp kosher salt
- 1 Tsp ground cinnamon
- 1/8 Tsp nutmeg
- Dash of cloves
- 3 - 4 Tsps Grated orange peel
- 1) 12oz Package vanilla chips

- Cream butter and sugars. Beat in egg.
- Combine dry Ingredients and add to Creamed Mixture.
- Stir in chips.

Direction

- Drop by rounded Tablespoons onto ungreased cookie sheet.
- Bake 350 for 12 - 14 Minutes or until lightly browned.
- Cool on wire racks.
- Makes about 3 dozen

47. Blueberry Almond Snickerdoodles Recipe

Serving: 16 | Prep: | Cook: 10mins | Ready in:

Ingredients

- 2 tablespoons butter, softened
- 2 tablespoons shortening
- 1/3 cup plus 2 tablespoons sugar, divided
- 1 egg
- 3/4 cup all-purpose flour
- 1/2 teaspoon cream of tartar
- 1/4 teaspoon baking soda
- 1/8 teaspoon salt
- 1/4 cup chopped almonds
- 1/4 cup dried blueberries
- 1/2 teaspoon ground cinnamon
- ICING:
- 1/4 cup confectioners' sugar
- 1 to 2 teaspoons 2% milk

Direction

- In a large bowl, cream the butter, shortening and 1/3 cup sugar until light and fluffy. Beat in egg.
- Combine the flour, cream of tartar, baking soda and salt;
- Gradually add to creamed mixture and mix well.

- Stir in almonds and blueberries.
- In a small bowl, combine cinnamon and remaining sugar.
- Shape dough into 1-1/2-in. balls; roll in cinnamon mixture. Place 2 in. apart on baking sheets coated with cooking spray.
- Bake at 350° for 10-12 minutes or until edges begin to brown.
- Cool for 2 minutes before removing from pans to wire racks to cool completely.
- For icing, combine confectioners' sugar and enough milk to achieve desired consistency. Drizzle over cookies.
- Store in an airtight container.
- Yield: about 1-1/4 dozen.

48. Blueberry Cheesecake Bars Recipe

Serving: 24 | Prep: | Cook: 30mins |Ready in:

Ingredients

- 6 tablespoons butter, melted
- 2 cups graham cracker crumbs
- 2 pkg. (8 oz.. each) cream cheese, softened
- 3/4 cup sugar
- 2 eggs, slightly beaten
- 1 teasppn vanilla
- 1 jar (10 oz.) blueberry jam or preserves
- 1 cup blueberries

Direction

- Preheat oven to 350-degrees
- Mix butter and graham crumbs in 13 x 9-inch baking pan.
- Press firmly onto bottom of pan.
- Refrigerate until ready to use.
- Brush with egg whites and bake. 5 to 10 Mins.
- Bake 30 minutes, or until slightly puffed.
- Cool completely in pan.
- Cut into 24 bars to serve.

- Store any leftover bars in tightly covered container in refrigerator up to 3 days. Also you can freeze up to a month.

49. Bodacious Chocolate Marshmallow Bars Recipe

Serving: 36 | Prep: | Cook: 20mins |Ready in:

Ingredients

- 3/4 cup butter
- 1-1/2 cups sugar
- 3 eggs
- 1 teaspoons vanilla extract
- 1-1/3 cups all purpose flour
- 3 tablespoons baking cocoa
- 1/2 teaspoons baking powder
- 1/2 teaspoon salt
- 1/2 cup chopped nuts, optional
- 4 cups miniature marshmallows
- Topping:
- 1-1/3 cup chocolate chips
- 1 cup peanut butter
- 3 tablespoons butter
- 2 cups crisp rice cereal

Direction

- In a mixing bowl, cream butter and sugar.
- Add eggs and vanilla; beat until fluffy.
- Combine flour, cocoa, baking powder and salt; add to creamed mixture.
- Stir in nuts if desired.
- Spread in a greased 15 x 10 x 1" pan. (I used a 9×13-inch pan)
- Bake at 350F for 15-18 minutes.
- Sprinkle marshmallows evenly over cake; return to oven for 2-3 minutes.
- Using a knife dipped in water, spread the melted marshmallows evenly over cake.
- Cool.
- For topping, combine chocolate chips, peanut butter and butter in a small saucepan.

- Cook over low heat, stirring constantly, until melted and well blended.
- Remove from heat; stir in cereal. Immediately spread over bars. Chill.

50. Boiled Cookies Recipe

Serving: 0 | Prep: | Cook: 10mins | Ready in:

Ingredients

- 2 cups white sugar
- 3 tablespoons unsweetened cocoa powder
- 1/2 cup margarine
- 1/2 cup milk
- 3 cups quick cooking oats
- 1/2 cup peanut butter
- 1 teaspoon vanilla extract

Direction

- 1. In a saucepan bring sugar, cocoa, margarine, and milk, to a rapid boil for 1 minute.
- 2. Add quick cooking oats, peanut butter, and vanilla; mix well.
- 3. Working quickly, drop by teaspoonful onto waxed paper, and let cool.

51. Bourbon Street Balls With Pecans Recipe

Serving: 30 | Prep: | Cook: | Ready in:

Ingredients

- 4 cups whole pecans or pecan halves
- 2 cup crushed or processed Nilla vanilla wafers
- 1 cup confectioners' sugar
- 4 jiggers (ounces) bourbon
- 3 tablespoons white Karo syrup
- butter, for fingertips

Direction

- Roughly chop the pecans in a food processor. Remove 2 cups and reserve. Finely grind the remaining pecans in the food processor.
- Combine ground pecans, Nella wafers, confectioners' sugar, bourbon, and syrup. Coat finger tips with softened butter to help you roll. Shape mixture into balls 1 1/2 inches in diameter using an ice cream scoop. Roll in chopped pecans. Arrange balls on a dessert platter and serve. Ask for help rolling. Four hands make very quick work of this dessert!
- NOTE: Store these in an air tight container and will save for 2-3 weeks. Longer they set, the more potent they get!

52. Breakfast Fig And Nut "cookies Recipe

Serving: 10 | Prep: | Cook: 14mins | Ready in:

Ingredients

- 3/4 cup packed brown sugar
- 1/4 cup butter, melted $
- 2 large eggs $
- 1/4 cup finely chopped dried figs
- 1/4 cup sweetened dried cranberries
- 1 teaspoon vanilla extract
- 1 cup all-purpose flour (about 4 1/2 ounces)
- 1/2 cup whole wheat flour (about 2 1/3 ounces)
- 1/2 cup unprocessed bran (about 1 ounce)
- 1/2 teaspoon baking soda
- 1/4 teaspoon ground cinnamon
- 1/4 teaspoon ground allspice
- 1/4 cup sliced almonds
- 2 teaspoons granulated sugar $

Direction

- Preheat oven to 350°.
- Combine first 3 ingredients in a large bowl. Stir in chopped figs, cranberries, and vanilla.

- Lightly spoon flours into dry measuring cups; level with a knife. Combine flours, bran, baking soda, cinnamon, and allspice, stirring with a whisk. Add flour mixture to egg mixture, stirring just until moist. Gently fold in almonds.
- Drop by level 1/4 cup measures 4 inches apart on 2 baking sheets lined with parchment paper. Sprinkle evenly with granulated sugar. Bake at 350° for 12 minutes or until almost set. Cool 2 minutes on pans. Remove from pans; cool completely on wire racks.
- Nutritional Information
- Amount per serving
- Calories: 211
- Calories from fat: 31%
- Fat: 7.1g
- Saturated fat: 3.3g
- Monounsaturated fat: 2.4g
- Polyunsaturated fat: 0.8g
- Protein: 4.5g
- Carbohydrate: 33.2g
- Fiber: 3.4g
- Cholesterol: 54mg
- Iron: 1.8mg
- Sodium: 115mg
- Calcium: 37mg

53. Buckeye Cookie Bars Recipe

Serving: 36 | Prep: | Cook: 25mins | Ready in:

Ingredients

- 1 Package chocolate cake mix (18 1/2 oz)
- 1/4 cup vegetable oil
- 1 egg
- 1 cup Chopped peanuts
- 1 Can sweetened condensed milk (14 oz)
- 1/2 cup peanut butter

Direction

- Preheat oven to 350F (325F for a glass dish).

- In large mixing bowl, combine cake mix, oil and egg; beat on medium speed until crumbly. Stir in peanuts.
- Reserving 1 1/2 cups crumb mixture, press remainder on bottom of greased 13x9-inch baking pan.
- In medium bowl, beat sweetened condensed milk with peanut butter until smooth; spread over prepared crust.
- Sprinkle with reserved crumb mixture.
- Bake 25 to 30 minutes or until set.
- Cool.
- Cut into bars. Store loosely covered at room temperature.

54. Buckeyes Recipe

Serving: 1 | Prep: | Cook: 50mins | Ready in:

Ingredients

- 2 cups peanut butter, organic non-sweetened if you have it is best
- 1 cup butter, softened, real of course (I wounder if 4oz of cream cheese would work for this instead??)
- 1/2 teaspoon vanilla extract
- 4 cups confectioners' sugar
- 4 cups semisweet chocolate chips, or chocolate bark, dark chocolate is great too

Direction

- In a large bowl, mix together the peanut butter, butter, vanilla and confectioners' sugar.
- The dough will look dry.
- Roll into 1 inch balls and place on a waxed paper-lined cookie sheet.
- Press a toothpick into the top of each ball (to be used later as the handle for dipping) and chill in freezer until firm, about 30 minutes.
- Melt chocolate chips in a double boiler or in a bowl set over a pan of barely simmering water.
- Stir frequently until smooth.

- Dip frozen peanut butter balls in chocolate holding onto the toothpick. Leave a small portion of peanut butter showing at the top to make them look like Buckeyes.
- Put back on the cookie sheet and refrigerate until serving.
- ~ ~ ~ ~ ~ ~ ~ ~
- A few other techniques that have helped others; you may wish to use one or more of these ideas. I add them here for your info, NOT as a must follow thing:
- *Chill the peanut butter mixture in the fridge 30 minutes before making the balls - this will help make a smoother, rounder buckeye.
- *Refrigerate the dough before rolling out the balls
- *Also, melt more chocolate than the recipe calls for so you have a good pool of chocolate to dip the ball into (you'll throw chocolate away, but it will make the product look better).
- *use real butter (well, duh!)
- *You can use one of those mini crock pots, dedicated to just chocolate melting, to melt the chocolate in. Keep it on low, the chocolate stays warm and when done you just put the lid on it and wait until you need it again.
- *DON'T take the balls out of the freezer until RIGHT before you are about to dip them. They will start to sweat after being out for a few minutes and this will keep the chocolate from sticking.
- *Definitely cut the sugar and sift it.
- *Add a tablespoon or two of shortening to the chocolate to help it stay a little firmer at room temperature; use semi-sweet chocolate as specified(I used a blend of milk choc and semi-sweet and it was too sweet).
- *Add some paraffin wax to the melted chocolate. The wax will thin out the chocolate and make it easier to dip. Plus, you won't use so much chocolate...this is especially helpful if you are making a double or triple batch like I do every year
- *Rolling the balls was very sticky, so I put powdered sugar on a paper plate and dipped both palms in after rolling each ball and it worked wonders; balls came out smooth.
- *Use an ice cream scoop to get a scoop of chocolate and then dip the balls in that. The ice cream scoop gets enough chocolate in it to make 3-4 small buckeyes and if it falls off the toothpick, it's not falling far! It also helps to get a full, nice covering of chocolate instead of having to roll around the ball to get the top partially covered. Then, you can use a shallower bowl instead of something too deep for the chocolate.
- *It works a lot better to cream the butter and p-nut butter together first and then add the sugar gradually. You need a dry dough, but if you just dump & stir as the recipe says it will be way too dry and the butter won't distribute correctly.
- * I don't recommend putting a tooth pick in every single one before chilling them. In fact, it works better NOT to because as the peanut butter cools it will pull away from the toothpick. I used ONE toothpick for my entire batch AFTER they chilled.
- *Cut the butter down to 1/4 cup (it really doesn't need butter at all to be delicious).
- *Take 5 balls out of the freezer at a time to dip in the melted mixture. You will get the hang of it after a while. There is definitely an art to dipping!
- *I used 1.5 bags of 12 ounce chips with a 1/2 4oz bar of shaved paraffin wax. Melt well. Paraffin wax is GREAT!
- *if you have choc left don't throw it out mix some cashews, or other nuts in the choc set on wax paper and let it harden ,then you have choc covered peanuts w/maybe a hint of peanut butter taste choc too expensive to throw out
- *Add a bit of shortening to the chocolate to give it a shine.
- * 3 cups sugar to 1 1/2 peanut butter are so much easier
- *chocolate bark to coat
- *add rice krispies
- *Use paraffin wax in your chocolate and whaala! It sticks!

- *dark chocolate is great too. You can also drizzle melted peanut butter chips on top or roll them into crushed peanuts. Make them in the gold 1 inch foil holders and place in some tins. They make great gifts to neighbors, friends, etc.
- *added 2 T shortening to chocolate and it coated nicely. I will do this from now on because I disliked other recipes that used paraffin wax
- *They're great frozen, and they last forever since they're so tasty and sweet it only takes a few to be satisfied.
- *don't freeze them either, just refrigerate until very firm. Freezing causes them to sweat.
- *MAIN THING: Close the toothpick hole!!! I hate to see them with the toothpick hole. Real buckeyes don't have a hole in the middle (unless it's got worms! LOL!)
- *altered the chocolate coating and used half milk and half semi-sweet chocolate chips and added about 2 tbsp. of butter and some heavy cream...at first my coating totally started to seize and I thought I'd wasted a ton of ingredients, but I just added some regular milk and it smoothed out
- *Use a 1 Tbsp. cookie scoop and did level sized scoops. I didn't bother to roll them, because I figured with the flat bottoms they would stand up better on the plate anyway.
- *Two suggestions that I will try the next time I make these. #1 - substitute 1 cup unsweetened cocoa for 1 cup confectioners' sugar & # 2 use unsweetened or perhaps bitter chocolate to coat these. If using bitter chocolate, let chocolate set & then sprinkle with icing sugar. This will make them look pretty too.
- *make sure your dough is cold, very cold or will be sticky when balling...use fruit baller to roll out even balls.

55. Burried Cherry Cookies Recipe

Serving: 46 | Prep: | Cook: 10mins | Ready in:

Ingredients

- 1 (10 ounce) jar maraschino cherries (42-48)
- 1/2 cup butter or margarine
- 1 cup sugar
- 1/4 teaspoon baking powder
- 1/4 teaspoon baking soda
- 1 egg
- 1 1/2 teaspoons vanilla
- 1/2 cup unsweetened cocoa powder
- 1 1/2 cups all purpose flour
- 1 (6 ounce) package (1 cup) semisweet chocolate pieces
- 1/2 cup sweetend condenesed milk or low-fat sweetened condensed milk

Direction

- Drain cherries, reserving juice. Halve any large cherries. In a medium mixing bowl beat butter with an electric mixer in medium to high speed for 30 seconds. Add the sugar, baking powder, baking soda, and 1/4 teaspoon of salt. Beat until combined, scraping sides of bowl. Beat in egg and vanilla until combined. Beat in cocoa powder and as much of the flour as you can with mixer. Stir in remaining flour using a wooden spoon.
- Shape dough into 1-inch balls. Place balls about 2 inches apart on an ungreased cookie sheet. Press your thumb into the center of each ball. Place a cherry in each center.
- For frosting, in a small saucepan combine chocolate pieces and sweetened condensed milk. Cook and stir over low heat until chocolate is melted. Stir in 4 teaspoons reserved cherry juice. Spoon 1 teaspoon frosting over each cherry, spreading to cover (frosting may be thinned with additional cherry juice if necessary). Bake in a 350 degrees oven for 10 minutes or until edges are firm. Cool 1 minute on cookie sheet. Transfer to a wire rack and let cool. This recipes requires the real goodness of chocolate so please don't substitute any non-chocolate product.

56. Buster Bar Dessert Recipe

Serving: 12 | Prep: | Cook: |Ready in:

Ingredients

- 1 lb. chocolate sandwhich cookies, crashed
- 1/2 cup butter or margarine
- 1/2 gallon of ice cream, softened slightly
- 1 1/2 cup Spanish peanuts
- 1/2 cup butter or margarine
- 2/3 cup chocolate chips
- 2/3 cup icing sugar
- 1 1/2 cup evaporated milk
- 1 tsp. vanilla

Direction

- Mix crushed cookies and 1/2 cup butter or margarine. Pat into 9 x 13 " pan. Spread softened ice cream over top of cookies patting down. Sprinkle peanuts over ice cream. Place in freezer.
- Mix 1/2 cup butter or margarine, sugar, chips and evaporated milk in a saucepan. Boil, stirring constantly, 5 to 8 minutes until thick. Cool and add vanilla. Once cool, pour over ice cream mixture.   Freeze. Remove from freezer a few minutes before serving to be able to cut it.

57. Butter Macadamia Nut Cookies Recipe

Serving: 12 | Prep: | Cook: 30mins |Ready in:

Ingredients

- butter Mac nut cookie Recipe
- 4 cups of regular flour
- 1 cup of powdered sugar
- 1 pound of butter, do not substitute margarine and have butter at room temperature.
- 2 cups or more of either raw or roasted macadamia nuts, chopped
- **Optional Flavors
- I add 2 tsp of lemon zest
- You can use either lemon, lime or orange zest.
- If you like coconut, add about a cup of sweetened shredded coconut or more depending on your preference. The more coconut, the chewier the cookie will be.
- 2 cups of chocolate chips, either semi-sweet or bittersweet
- Chopped pecans, walnuts, brazil nuts, hazel nuts or even peanuts.
- (Bittersweet chips and orange zest or lemon zest make a fabulous cookie!)
- And of course, you can dip your cookie in chocolate! Chocoholics, Unite! Melt 1 cup of chips with 1 tsp of butter in the microwave for one minute, stir and dip the cooled cookie bars into the chocolate and lay on wax paper or aluminum to dry. You can even dip the dipped chocolate into some finely chopped nuts or coconute for a fancier cookie.

Direction

- Beat the butter until it's soft.
- Add the sugar and beat until it's very smooth.
- Add the nuts and zest and blend well.
- Using a large baking pan, either roll out the dough to 1/2 an inch thick or pat it directly on to the pan using your hands. (I use the "release" aluminum foil or a large silicone baking mat.)
- You can flour your baking pan if you don't have the foil or a baking mat but do not butter your pan.
- Bake this at 300 degrees for about 30 minutes or until firm.
- When the sides start to turn to a golden brown, the rest of the dough is done.
- Score and cut your squares about five minutes after removing dough from the oven.

- If you're making individual cookies, cut the shapes you wish after mixing and bake until each cookie is a very light color. You can make the tiny cookies too that you find in Hawaii but watch them carefully in the oven.

58. Butter Tart Squares Recipe

Serving: 9 | Prep: | Cook: 40mins | Ready in:

Ingredients

- 1/2 cup of butter
- 1/3 cup of white sugar
- 1 cup of all purpose flour
- 2 eggs beaten
- 2 tbsp of flour
- 1/2 tsp of vanilla
- 1 1/2 cup of raisins (or use Cranraisins for a twist)
- 1 cup of brown sugar
- 1/2 tsp of baking powder pinch of salt
- 1/2 tsp of grated lemon rind (add with Cranraisins, nice punch)

Direction

- Blend first three ingredients until it is a crumb texture.
- Spread in the bottom of an 8 x 8 inch pan, ungreased.
- Bake 15 minutes at 350 degrees.
- Mix filling; spread over base.
- Bake another 25 minutes.
- Cut when cool.

59. CARAMEL SQUARES Recipe

Serving: 8 | Prep: | Cook: 25mins | Ready in:

Ingredients

- 2 C. graham cracker crumbs (about 20 graham crackers)
- 1 can sweetened condensed milk
- 6-oz. package of butterscotch chips
- 1 C. chopped nuts, lightly toasted

Direction

- Preheat oven to 325°
- Grease and flour 9-inch square pan.
- Combine all ingredients and spread in pan.
- Bake for 20 to 25 minutes.
- Cut into squares while still warm.

60. CARROT COOKIES Recipe

Serving: 18 | Prep: | Cook: 20mins | Ready in:

Ingredients

- 1 cup butter, softened
- 3/4 cup sugar
- 1 cup mashed, cooked carrots
- 1/2 teaspoon lemon extract
- 1/2 teaspoon almond extract
- 2 cups flour
- 2 teaspoons baking powder
- 1/4 teaspoon salt
- 1/2 cup chopped nuts
- 1/2 cup golden raisins

Direction

- Beat butter, sugar, mashed carrots and extracts together until well-blended.
- Combine flour, baking powder and salt. Add to creamed mixture, and mix well.
- Stir in nuts and raisins.
- Drop by heaping teaspoonfuls onto a greased cookie sheet.
- Bake at 350 degrees for 20-25 minutes until lightly golden.

61. CLARK BAR COOKIES Recipe

Serving: 1 | Prep: | Cook: | Ready in:

Ingredients

- 4 c. crushed graham crackers
- 2 c. peanut butter
- 12 oz. pkg. chocolate chips
- 1 can Eagle Brand milk
- 1 c. butter, melted
- 2 1/2 c. powdered sugar

Direction

- Mix by hand the graham crackers crumbs, peanut butter, powdered sugar and butter.
- Press into jelly roll pan.
- Melt chocolate chips and milk over low heat. Pour over graham cracker mixture. Refrigerate.

62. Candy Bar Cake Recipe

Serving: 12 | Prep: | Cook: 45mins | Ready in:

Ingredients

- 1 box milk chocolate or German chocolate cake mix
- 1 can condensed sweetened milk
- 1 bottle caramel ice cream topping
- tub of Cool Whip
- Heath Toffee bits

Direction

- Bake cake as directed.
- When done, poke holes into cake about 1 inch apart.
- While still warm pour condensed milk into holes.
- Then pour caramel into the holes.
- When cake is completely cooled, spread Cool Whip on top of cake and sprinkle with toffee bits.

- Keep refrigerated.

63. Candy Cane Shortbread Recipe

Serving: 44 | Prep: | Cook: 30mins | Ready in:

Ingredients

- 2 cups butter, softened
- 1 cup granulated sugar
- 1 tsp peppermint extract
- 3½ cups all-purpose flour
- 1 cup rice flour
- 3/4 cup crushed candy cane

Direction

- Beat butter until almost white.
- Add sugar and peppermint extract and beat until fluffy.
- In another bowl, stir together all-purpose and rice flours.
- Add to butter mixture in 3 additions and stir to combine well.
- Stir in crushed candy canes.
- Preheat oven to 275°F
- Gather dough together and divide into 4 discs.
- Roll each disc between 2 pieces of waxed or parchment paper to a generous 1/4-inch thickness.
- Cut out cookies using 3-inch round cookie cutter (or whatever shape you prefer) and place on parchment-paper-lined baking sheet.
- Freeze for 15 minutes or until firm.
- Repeat with remaining dough, re-rolling scraps.
- Bake 1 tray at a time on centre rack of the oven for about 30 minutes or until firm to the touch.
- Let cool in pan on rack for 5 minutes.
- Remove cookies to cooling rack and let cool completely.
- Tip
- There are a couple of ways to crush your candy canes. For this recipe it is best to use a food processor on pulse to get crushed pieces

that have some fine powder and smaller pieces throughout. Or, place candy canes in a plastic storage bag, and gently break with a small hammer or meat tenderizer.

64. Caramel Heavenlies Recipe

Serving: 48 | Prep: | Cook: 15mins |Ready in:

Ingredients

- 16 graham crackers
- 2 cups miniature marshmallows
- 3/4 cup butter
- 1 teaspoon vanilla extract
- 3/4 cup brown sugar
- 2 cups sliced almonds
- 2 cups flaked coconut

Direction

- Preheat oven to 350 degrees F.
- Line a 10x15 inch jellyroll pan with aluminum foil.
- Arrange graham crackers to cover the bottom of the prepared pan. In a small saucepan, combine the butter and brown sugar.
- Cook over medium heat, stirring occasionally until smooth. Remove from the heat and stir in the vanilla.
- Sprinkle the marshmallows over the graham cracker crust.
- Pour the butter mixture evenly over the graham crackers and marshmallows.
- Sprinkle the coconut and almonds evenly over the marshmallows.
- Bake for 14 minutes in the preheated oven, until coconut and almonds are toasted.
- Allow the bars to cool completely before cutting into triangles.
- Store at room temperature in an airtight container.

65. Caramel Oatmeal Bars Recipe

Serving: 18 | Prep: | Cook: 30mins |Ready in:

Ingredients

- 3/4 cup shortening (Crisco butter or 3/4 stick Crisco butter shortening Sticks)
- 1 1/2 cups quick oats, uncooked
- 3/4 cup brown sugar, firmly packed
- 1/2 cup all-purpose flour, plus
- 3 tablespoons flour
- 1/2 cup whole wheat flour
- 1/2 teaspoon baking soda
- 1/4 teaspoon ground cinnamon
- 1 1/3 cups milk chocolate chips
- 1/2 cup walnuts, chopped
- 1 (12 1/2 ounce) jar caramel ice cream topping, Smuckers

Direction

- HEAT oven to 350°F
- Coat a 9 x 9 x 2-inch baking pan with no-stick cooking spray.
- COMBINE shortening, oats, brown sugar, 1/2 cup all-purpose flour, whole wheat flour, baking soda and cinnamon in large bowl.
- With an electric mixer at low speed, blend until mixture resembles coarse crumbs.
- Reserve 1/2 cup for topping. Press remaining crumbs into prepared pan.
- BAKE 10 minutes. Remove from oven.
- SPRINKLE chocolate chips and nuts over crust.
- Stir together caramel topping and 3 tablespoons flour until well blended.
- Drizzle over chocolate chips and nuts.
- Top with reserved 1/2 cup crumbs.
- RETURN to oven.
- Bake an additional 20 to 25 minutes or until golden brown.
- While still warm, run a knife around the outside edge of pan.
- Cool completely on rack.
- CUT into squares.

66. Caramel Walnut Dream Bars Recipe

Serving: 16 | Prep: | Cook: 35mins | Ready in:

Ingredients

- 1 box yellow cake mix
- 3 tablespoons butter softened
- 1 egg
- 14 ounces sweetened condensed milk
- 1 egg
- 1 teaspoon pure vanilla extract
- 1/2 cup walnuts finely ground
- 1/2 cup finely ground toffee bits

Direction

- Preheat oven to 350. Prepare rectangular cake pan with cooking spray then set aside. Combine cake mix, butter and one egg in a mixing bowl then mix until crumbly. Press mixture onto bottom of prepared pan then set aside. In another mixing bowl combine milk, remaining egg, extract, walnuts and toffee bits. Mix well and pour over base in pan. Bake for 35 minutes.

67. Cashew Triangles Recipe

Serving: 12 | Prep: | Cook: 20mins | Ready in:

Ingredients

- 1/2 cup butter softened
- 1/4 cup granulated sugar
- 1/4 cup packed brown sugar
- 1/2 teaspoon vanilla
- 1 egg separated
- 1 cup all purpose flour
- 1/8 teaspoon salt
- 1 teaspoon water
- 1 cup chopped salted cashews

- 1 ounce unsweetened chocolate melted and cooled

Direction

- Preheat oven to 350.
- Mix butter, sugars, vanilla and egg yolk in medium bowl then stir in flour and salt.
- Press dough in ungreased rectangular pan with floured hands.
- Beat egg white and water then brush over dough.
- Sprinkle with cashews and press lightly into dough.
- Bake 25 minutes or until light brown then cool 10 minutes and cut into 3" squares.
- Cut each square diagonally in half then immediately remove from pan and cool.
- Drizzle with chocolate then allow to stand 2 hours to allow chocolate to set.

68. Cheese Cake Cooky Squares Recipe

Serving: 16 | Prep: | Cook: 45mins | Ready in:

Ingredients

- 5 tablespoons butter, softened
- 1/3 cup brown sugar, packed
- 1 cup flour
- 1/2 cup sugar
- 1 (8 ounce) packet cream cheese, softened
- 1 egg
- 2 tablespoons milk
- 1 tablespoon lemon juice
- 1/2 teaspoon vanilla

Direction

- Preheat oven to 350F.
- In a medium bowl blend thoroughly butter, brown sugar and flour with a fork until mixture resembles coarse crumbs.
- Put 1 cup of the mixture aside for topping.

- Press remaining mixture into an 8x8x2 inch baking dish sprayed lightly with cooking spray; bake for 15 minutes.
- In another bowl combine sugar and cream cheese, mixing until smooth.
- Thoroughly beat in egg, milk, lemon juice and vanilla.
- Spread over the baked crust and sprinkle with remaining brown sugar mixture.
- Bake for 25 minutes.
- Let cool, then chill for at least 1 hour.
- Cut into 16 squares; serve.

69. Cheesecake Bar Cookies Recipe

Serving: 36 | Prep: | Cook: 25mins |Ready in:

Ingredients

- 9 sq. graham crackers, finely crushed
- 1/2 C. flour
- 1/2 C. chopped walnuts
- 1/4 C. sugar
- 1/2 C. butter, melted
- 1 (8 oz.) pkg. cream cheese, softened
- 1/3 C. sugar
- 1 egg
- 1 Tbs. lemon juice
- 2 Tbs. finely crushed graham cracker

Direction

- Stir together first 4 ingredients add melted butter, mix until crumbly.
- Pat into ungreased 9x9x2 baking dish.
- Bake at 350°F for 10 minutes.
- Blend cream cheese and sugar.
- Add egg and lemon juice.
- Mix well.
- Pour over baked layer.
- Bake for 20 to 25 minutes.
- Sprinkle with cracker crumbs.
- Cool and cut in squares.
- Yields 3 dozen. Store in refrigerator.

70. Cherry Almond Cookies Recipe

Serving: 12 | Prep: | Cook: 15mins |Ready in:

Ingredients

- 1 cup butter
- 1 cup brown sugar
- 1/2 cup white sugar
- 2 eggs
- 2 tablespoons milk
- 2 teaspoons almond extract
- 2-1/2 cups rolled oats
- 1-3/4 cups flour
- 1/4 teaspoon salt
- 1 teaspoon baking soda
- 1 cup sliced almonds
- 1 cup dried cherries
- 1/2 cup dried coconut

Direction

- Cream butter then gradually add sugars until fluffy.
- Beat in eggs, milk and extract then add flour, salt and baking soda.
- Stir in oats, cherries, almonds and coconut then bake at 350 for 12 minutes.

71. Cherry Bonbon Cookies Recipe

Serving: 24 | Prep: | Cook: 20mins |Ready in:

Ingredients

- 24 maraschino cherries undrained
- 1/2 cup butter softened
- 3/4 cup sifted powdered sugar
- 1-1/2 cups all purpose flour
- 1/8 teaspoon salt
- 2 tablespoons light cream
- 1 teaspoon vanilla extract
- powdered sugar

- Cherry Glaze:
- 2 tablespoons butter melted
- 1 cup sifted powdered sugar
- 1/4 cup reserved cherry juice
- red food coloring

Direction

- Drain cherries reserving 1/4 cup juice for glaze then set aside.
- Beat butter at medium speed with an electric mixer until creamy.
- Gradually add 3/4 cup powdered sugar beating well.
- Stir in flour and next 3 ingredients then shape into 24 balls.
- Press each ball around a cherry covering completely then place on ungreased cookie sheets.
- Bake at 350 for 20 minutes then remove to wire racks to cool completely.
- Sprinkle with powdered sugar and drizzle with cherry glaze.
- To make glaze combine first 3 ingredients then add food coloring.
- Place in small plastic bag and seal.
- To drizzle snip a tiny hole at one corner of bag and gently squeeze bag.

72. Cherry Cream Gelatin Squares Recipe

Serving: 15 | Prep: | Cook: |Ready in:

Ingredients

- GELATIN:
- 6 oz. pkg. cherry flavor gelatin
- 2 cups boiling water
- 1 cup cold water
- 2 Tbs. lemon juice
- 1/2 tsp. almond extract
- 21 oz. can cherry pie filling
- TOPPING:

- 1/2 cup sugar
- 1/2 cup sour cream
- 8 oz. pkg. cream cheese, softened

Direction

- In large bowl, dissolve gelatine in boiling water. Stir in cold water, lemon juice, almond extract and pie filling. Pour into ungreased 13x9 baking dish. Refrigerate until firm.
- In small bowl, combine topping ingredients, beat until smooth. Carefully spread over firm gelatine.
- Refrigerate until ready to serve.

73. Cherry Nut Bars Recipe

Serving: 16 | Prep: | Cook: 45mins |Ready in:

Ingredients

- 2 cup flour
- 2 cup oatmeal
- 1 1/2 cup sugar
- 1/2 cup chopped pecans
- 1 tsp baking soda
- 1 1/4 c butter, melted
- 21 oz can cherry pie filling
- 1 c mini marshmallows

Direction

- In 3 qt. mixer bowl, combine flour, oats, sugar, pecans, soda and butter.
- Mix at low speed scraping sides until crumbly, 2 - 3 minutes.
- Reserve 1 1/2 cup crumb mixture for topping.
- Press crumb mixture evenly into 13x9x2 pan.
- Bake near center of oven for 12 to 15 min. or until lightly browned at edges.
- Gently spoon pie filling evenly over crust, sprinkle with marshmallows and crumb mixture.
- Return to oven for 25 -35 minutes or until lightly browned.

- Cool and cut into bars.

74. Cherry Squares Recipe

Serving: 10 | Prep: | Cook: 45mins | Ready in:

Ingredients

- 1/2 cup butter
- 1/2 cup margarine
- 1-3/4 cups sugar
- 4 eggs
- 1 tsp. vanilla
- 1/2 tsp. almond flavouring
- 1/2 tsp. soda
- 1-1/2 tsp. baking powder
- 3 cups flour
- 1/2 tsp. salt
- 1 can cherry pie filling

Direction

- Cream the shortening and sugar.
- Beat well.
- Add eggs, one at a time.
- Add vanilla and almond flavouring.
- Sift the dry ingredients together and add gradually to creamed mixture.
- Save back a little more than one cup of batter.
- Spread the rest in an 11 x 17 inch greased pan.
- Spread the pie filling over the batter.
- Spoon the remaining one cup of batter in small islands over the cherry layer.
- Bake at 350 degrees F for 40-45 minutes.
- Sprinkle top with powdered sugar.
- Cut into squares when cool.

75. Chewy Coconut Cookies Recipe

Serving: 36 | Prep: | Cook: 8mins | Ready in:

Ingredients

- 2 cups all-purpose flour
- 2/3 cup sugar
- 3/4 teaspoon baking soda
- 1/4 teaspoon salt
- 1/3 cup dark corn syrup
- 3 tablespoons vegetable oil
- 1 teaspoon vanilla extract
- 1 teaspoon coconut extract
- 2 egg whites
- 1/3 cup coconut - flaked
- vegetable cooking spray
- 2 tablespoons coconut - flaked and toasted

Direction

- Combine first 4 ingredients in a large bowl; stir well. In a small bowl combine corn syrup, oil, extracts, and egg whites; stir well. Add corn syrup mixture to dry ingredients, stirring just until dry ingredients are moistened. Stir in 1/3 cup coconut.
- Drop dough by level tablespoons onto baking sheets coated with cooking spray. Sprinkle toasted coconut over cookies.
- Bake at 350° F. for 8 minutes; let cool on pans 1 minute. Remove from pans; let cool completely on wire racks.

76. Chock Full O Chips Cookie Bars Recipe

Serving: 36 | Prep: | Cook: 30mins | Ready in:

Ingredients

- 1 cup butter
- 2 large eggs
- 1 1/2 cups packed brown sugar
- 2 tablespoons coffee flavored liqueur, or milk
- 1 teaspoon vanilla
- 2 cups flour
- 1 teaspoon baking powder
- 1/4 teaspoon baking soda
- 1/4 teaspoon salt

- 3/4 cup double fudge chocolate chips
- 3/4 cup peanut butter chips
- 3/4 cup white chocolate chips
- 3/4 cup toffee pieces

Direction

- Preheat oven to 350.
- Coat a 9 x 13 baking pan with cooking spray.
- In a large mixing bowl, using an electric mixer on medium high speed, combine butter, eggs and brown sugar and beat until creamy.
- Add coffee flavored liqueur and vanilla and mix well.
- Reduce speed to low and gradually add in flour, baking powder, baking soda and salt. Mix until well blended. Fold in chips and toffee pieces.
- Stir until all chips are evenly distributed in dough.
- Spread dough in pan and bake 30 to 35 minutes. Let cool before cutting into bars.

77. Chocolate Banana Cookies Recipe

Serving: 10 | Prep: | Cook: 1hours |Ready in:

Ingredients

- 1 ripen banana
- 250g flour
- 1 tsp baking powder
- 1 tbsp cocoa powder
- 100g sugar
- 2 tsp vanilla sugar
- pinch of salt
- 100g unsalted butter [room temperature]

Direction

- Mash banana with a fork.
- Sift the flour, cocoa powder and baking powder.

- Add sugar, vanilla sugar, salt, cubed butter and mashed banana.
- Mix with a food mixer until it becomes like big crumbs.
- Then knead it with hands until smooth and even.
- Form 4cm [1.6 inch] diameter balls, flatten a little and divide into 6 pieces [triangular]
- Place them on a baking paper and bake in preheated oven [180C - 356F] for 15-20 minutes.
- When they are baked, let them cool in a baking tray for 5 minutes and then place them on a cooling rack.
- Dust with caster sugar.

78. Chocolate Bar Nut Brownies Recipe

Serving: 24 | Prep: | Cook: 35mins |Ready in:

Ingredients

- 1 (17 5/8 ounce) package walnut brownie mix (Duncan Hines)
- vegetable oil
- water
- eggs
- 3 (8 Oz) Symphony chocolate bars with almond and Toffee (a must)
- 1/2 Cup Chopped walnuts (optional)

Direction

- Prepare the brownie mix according to package directions.
- Add the Chopped Walnuts to the mix.
- Line a 13 by 9-inch cake pan with aluminum foil and spray with vegetable oil cooking spray. Spoon in half of the brownie batter and smooth with a spatula or the back of a spoon. Place the candy bars side by side on top of the batter. (Do not break) Cover with the remaining batter.

- Bake according to package directions. Let cool completely, then lift from the pan using the edges of the foil. This makes it easy to cut the brownies into squares.

79. Chocolate Carmal Bars Recipe

Serving: 12 | Prep: | Cook: 25mins | Ready in:

Ingredients

- 1 - pkg of Carmels
- 1 cup plus of chocolate chips
- 1/2 cup evaporated milk (I even use fat free but either way is good)
- 3/4 cup butter
- 1 German chocolate cake mix (Betty Crocker)
- 1/2 cup of evaporated milk

Direction

- In saucepan melt caramels with 1/2 cup of evaporate milk stirring constantly then set aside.
- Mix cake mix with melted butter and other 1/2 cup of evaporated milk (you can add nuts-optional).
- Press 1/2 mixture in cake pan and bake at 350 for 6 minutes.
- Sprinkle chocolate chips over top of partially baked cake mix and pour the caramel on top of that. (You can use butterscotch and peanut butter chips if you want to also)
- Sprinkle the remaining cake mixture in clumps over the top and bake at 350 for another 15-18 minutes.
- Cool and cut.

80. Chocolate Chip Oatmeal Cookies Recipe

Serving: 0 | Prep: | Cook: 15mins | Ready in:

Ingredients

- 2 cups sifted flour
- 1 tsp baking powder
- 1 tsp baking soda
- 1/2 tsp salt
- 1 cup shortening
- 1 cup brown sugar, packed
- 1 cup sugar
- 2 eggs
- 1 tsp vanilla
- 2 cups quick-cooking oats
- 1 (12 oz.) pkg. semisweet chocolate pieces
- 1/2 cup chopped walnuts

Direction

- Sift together the flour, baking powder, baking soda, and salt
- Set aside
- Cream together the shortening, brown sugar, and sugar in a bowl until light and fluffy, using an electric mixer at medium speed
- Add the eggs, one at a time
- Beat well after each addition
- Blend in the vanilla
- Gradually stir the dry ingredients into the creamed mixture.
- Blend well
- Stir in the oats, chocolate pieces, and the walnuts.
- Drop the mixture by teaspoonfuls, about 2 inches apart, onto greased
- Baking sheets.
- Bake in 350 F for 12 to 15 minutes, or until golden brown
- Remove from the baking sheets
- Cool on wire racks

81. Chocolate Chip Cookie Makeover Recipe

Serving: 36 | Prep: | Cook: 15mins | Ready in:

Ingredients

- 1-1/2 cups all-purpose flour
- 3/4 teaspoon baking powder
- 1/4 teaspoon baking soda
- 1/2 teaspoon salt
- 1 cup packed dark brown sugar
- 1/4 cup unsalted butter softened
- 1 teaspoon vanilla extract
- 1/4 cup fat free sour cream
- 1 large egg
- 3/4 cup quick cooking rolled oats
- 1/2 cup miniature chocolate chips

Direction

- Preheat oven to 350.
- Spray 2 large baking sheets with non-stick spray.
- Combine flour, baking powder, baking soda and salt in a bowl then set aside.
- With an electric mixer on medium high beat brown sugar, butter and vanilla until blended.
- Stir in oats and chocolate chips.
- Drop dough by level tablespoonfuls onto baking sheets 1" apart making a total of 36 cookies.
- Dip bottom of a glass in flour and press floured glass against each mound.
- Bake 1 sheet at a time until lightly browned about 12 minutes.
- Transfer to racks and cool then repeat with remaining cookies.

82. Chocolate Chip Cookies Recipe

Serving: 60 | Prep: | Cook: 12mins | Ready in:

Ingredients

- 1 1/2 cups LAND O LAKES® butter, softened
- 1 1/4 cups firmly packed brown sugar
- 1 cup sugar
- 2 eggs

- 1 tablespoon vanilla
- 3 3/4 cups all-purpose flour
- 1 cup uncooked quick-cooking oats
- 2 teaspoons baking soda
- 1 teaspoon salt
- 2 cups real semi-sweet chocolate chips

Direction

- Heat oven to 350°F.
- Combine butter, brown sugar and sugar in large bowl. Beat at medium speed, scraping bowl often, until creamy.
- Add eggs and vanilla; continue beating until well mixed.
- Reduce speed to low; add all remaining cookie ingredients except chocolate chips.
- Beat until well mixed.
- Stir in chocolate chips.
- Drop dough by rounded tablespoonful, 2 inches apart, onto ungreased cookie sheets.
- Bake for 10 to 12 minutes or until very lightly browned. Let stand 1 minute; remove from cookie sheets.
- *Substitute 1 1/2 cups candy-coated chocolate pieces or 2 (4-ounce) bars milk chocolate, cut into small chunks or 1 1/2 cups raisins.
- VARIATIONS:
- Cocoa Chocolate Chip Cookies: Prepare cookies as directed above except omit quick-cooking oats and substitute 1/2 cup unsweetened cocoa.
- Peanutty Chocolate Chip Cookies: Prepare cookies as directed above except omit quick-cooking oats and substitute 1 cup peanut butter.
- Easy Chocolate Chip Bars: Prepare cookies as directed above. Spread dough into lightly greased 15x10x1-inch jelly-roll pan. Bake for 25 to 30 minutes or until toothpick inserted in center comes out clean. 48 bars.
- Recipe Tip
- If cookies spread too much during baking, chill dough 1 hour. If cookies still spread too much, stir in 1 to 2 tablespoons flour.
- Nutrition Facts (1 cookie): Calories: 130, Fat: 7g, Cholesterol: 20mg, Sodium: 130mg,

Carbohydrates: 18g, Dietary Fiber: 0g, Protein: 2g

83. Chocolate Chip Cookies Mix In A Jar Recipe

Serving: 12 | Prep: | Cook: 10mins |Ready in:

Ingredients

- This is a mix in a jar sort of recipe so the rest of the ingredients will be listed in the directions:
- 1 ¾ cups all purpose flour
- ¾ teaspoon baking soda
- ¾ teaspoon salt
- 1 ½ cups or 9 ounces semi-sweet chocolate chips
- ¾ cup packed brown sugar
- ½ cup granulated sugar
- Combine flour, baking soda, and salt in a small bowl. Place flour mixture in 1 quart canning jar. Place chocolate chips in next followed by brown sugar and then white sugar.
- It is helpful to tap jar on a lightly padded surface.
- To top the jar off making it more decorative cut a 9 inch circle from fabric of your choice, fastening in place with a rubber band. You may wish to add raffia or ribbon bow to cover the rubber band.

Direction

- Create and attach a card with the following directions:
- ¾ cup or 1 ½ sticks butter or margarine
- 1 large egg
- ¾ teaspoon vanilla
- ½ nuts optional
- Preheat oven to 375°F.
- Beat ¾ cup softened butter or margarine, 1 large egg and ¾ teaspoon vanilla extract in large mixer bowl until blended.

- Add cookie mix and ½ cup chopped nuts (optional); mix well, breaking up any clumps.
- Drop by rounded tablespoon onto un-greased baking sheets.
- Bake for 9 to 11 minutes or until golden brown.
- Cool on baking sheets for 2 minutes; remove to wire racks to cool completely. Makes about 2 dozen cookies.

84. Chocolate Chip Cream Cheese Cookies Recipe

Serving: 1 | Prep: | Cook: 10mins |Ready in:

Ingredients

- 1/4 c. butter
- 1 (8 oz.) pkg. cream cheese
- 1 egg
- 1/4 tsp. vanilla
- 1 pkg. (2 layer) yellow cake mix
- 1 (8 oz) pkg. chocolate chips
- 1/2 c. chopped nuts

Direction

- Cream butter & cheese until light & fluffy.
- Beat in egg & vanilla & add the cake mix a little at a time until all had been added & is smooth.
- Stir in nuts & chips.
- Bake at 375 F. for 10 to 12 min.

85. Chocolate Chip Meltaways Recipe

Serving: 40 | Prep: | Cook: 12mins |Ready in:

Ingredients

- 1 cup butter or oleo softened

- 1 cup vegetable oil
- 1 cup sugar
- 1 cup confectioners sugar, sifted
- 2 eggs
- 4 cups flour
- 1 teaspoon baking soda
- 1 teaspoon cream of tarter
- 1 teaspoon salt
- 1 teaspoon vanilla
- 12oz package semi-sweet chocolate chips
- additional sugar

Direction

- Combine first five ingredients in a large bowl. Beat until smooth.
- Combine flour, soda, creams of tarter, and salt. Add to butter mixture. Beat until smooth.
- Stir in vanilla and chocolate chips. Shape mixture into 1" balls. Roll in granulated sugar.
- Put 2" apart on ungreased cookie sheets and bake at 395 degrees for 10-12 minutes. Cool.
- Can wrap well and freeze.

86. Chocolate Chip N Banana Drop Cookies Recipe

Serving: 36 | Prep: | Cook: 12mins | Ready in:

Ingredients

- 1 1/2 cups all-purpose flour
- 1/4 teaspoon baking soda
- 1/4 teaspoon salt
- 3/4 cup unsalted butter, room temperature
- 2/3 cup granulated sugar
- 1/3 cup packed brown sugar
- 1 egg
- 1 medium overripe banana
- 2 teaspoons vanilla extract
- 1 cup old-fashioned rolled oats
- 1 cup (6 ounces) milk chocolate chips

Direction

- Preheat oven to 350 degrees.
- In a small bowl, combine the flour, baking soda and salt; set aside.
- In a mixing bowl, cream the butter with the sugars.
- Add the egg, banana and vanilla; beat until smooth.
- Beat in the flour mixture.
- Stir in the oats and chocolate chips.
- Drop the batter by large spoonfuls 2 inches apart onto non-stick baking sheets (or line the sheets with parchment paper).
- Bake for 10 to 14 minutes, until lightly browned and almost firm when pressed in the center.
- Remove the entire baking sheet to a wire rack to cool for 2 to 3 minutes, then transfer the cookies to the rack to completely cool.

87. Chocolate Chippers Recipe

Serving: 0 | Prep: | Cook: 15mins | Ready in:

Ingredients

- 1 cup shortening
- 1 cup white sugar
- 1/2 cup brown sugar
- 2 eggs
- 2 tsp vanilla
- 2 1/2 cups flour
- 1/2 tsp salt
- 1 tsp baking soda
- 2 cups chocolate chips

Direction

- Cream shortening, sugars, eggs, and vanilla until light and fluffy.
- Mix dry ingredients, then add to the wet, mixing well.
- Add chocolate chips.
- On greased baking sheet, bake at 370° for 10-12 min.
- Enjoy!

88. Chocolate Cookie Turtles Recipe

Serving: 24 | Prep: | Cook: 13mins | Ready in:

Ingredients

- 2 cups (120) pecan halves
- 20 unwrapped caramels
- 1 package (18 oz) refrigerated chocolate chip cookie dough
- 2 tbsp. milk

Direction

- Soak the pecans for 5 minutes in water to soften.
- Arrange 5 pecans on an ungreased baking sheet (4 for legs, 1 for head), leaving a 1-inch circle in the center.
- Shape level tbsp. of cookie dough into a ball and place over the circle between the pecans, pressing onto the nuts.
- Repeat with the remaining pecans and dough, placing the turtles 2 inches apart on the baking sheets.
- Bake in a preheated oven (350 degrees) for 11 to 13 minutes or until the edges are crisp. Let stand for 1 minute and then remove to wire racks to cool.
- Microwave the caramels and milk on high power for 1 1/2 minutes; stir. Microwave at additional 10-sec intervals until melted.
- Drizzle mixture over turtles.
- ENJOY!!

89. Chocolate Covered Cherry Cookies Recipe

Serving: 48 | Prep: | Cook: 10mins | Ready in:

Ingredients

- 1 and 1/2 cups flour
- 1/2 cup cocoa powder
- 1/4 teasp. salt
- 1/4 teasp. baking powder
- 1/4 teasp. baking soda
- 1/2 cup butter,softened
- 1 cup sugar
- 1 egg
- 1 and 1/2 teasp. vanilla extract,pure
- 1 (10oz) jar maraschino cherries(about 48)
- 1 6 (oz) package semisweet chocolate chips(I use milk chocolate chips)
- 1/2 cup Eagle Brand milk

Direction

- In large bowl stir together flour, cocoa, salt, baking powder, soda
- Set aside
- In mixer bowl beat together butter, sugar on low, till fluffy
- Add egg and vanilla, beat well
- Gradually add dry ingredients to creamed mixture, beat till well blended.
- Shape dough into 1 in. balls
- Place onto ungreased cookie sheet
- Press down center of dough with thumb
- Drain maraschino cherries, reserving juice
- Place a cherry in the center of each cookie
- In small sauce pan combine chocolate chips and Eagle Brand, heat until melted
- Stir in 4 teaspoon of the reserved cherry juice
- Spoon about 1 teaspoon frosting over cherry, making sure to cover all of the cherry
- Many thin frosting with a little more cherry juice,
- Bake in a 350-degree oven for 10 minutes
- Remove to wire rack
- Cool

90. Chocolate Dipped Fruit Filled Cookies Recipe

Serving: 16 | Prep: | Cook: | Ready in:

Ingredients

- 1 container (7 oz.) BAKER'S Real milk Dipping chocolate or other company of your choice
- 16 fig Newtons or other fruit Chewy cookie
- **Option** You can use a darker chocolate or even white chocolate to make a design on the cookies in layers!**

Direction

- MELT chocolate as directed on package; stir until smooth.
- DIP each cookie into chocolate, completely coating bottom half of each cookie.
- Place in single layer on wax paper-covered baking sheet.
- REFRIGERATE 15 min. or until chocolate is firm.
- SERVE with Milk for the kids or an afternoon Tea or Coffee for Adults!

91. Chocolate Divine Pecan Bars Recipe

Serving: 24 | Prep: | Cook: 25mins | Ready in:

Ingredients

- 2 sticks unsalted butter, softened
- 2 cups flour
- 1/2 cup sugar
- 1/4 teaspoon salt
- 1-1/2 cups semi sweet chocolate chips
- 1 (14 ounce) can Eagle Brand milk
- 1-1/2 teaspoons vanilla
- 1 cup pecans, chopped
- 1/2 cup semi sweet chocolate chips

Direction

- In large mixer bowl, cream butter
- Add flour, sugar and salt
- Beat until crumbly
- Press *2 cups* mixture into a greased 9X13 inch baking pan, reserving the remaining crumbs
- Bake at 350 degrees for 10 minutes or until golden brown
- Combine 1-1/2 cups chocolate chips, condensed milk in saucepan
- Heat until chocolate is melted, stirring constantly
- Stir in vanilla
- Spread over hot crust
- Combine the pecans, 1/2 cup chocolate chips and *reserved crumbs*
- Sprinkle this over the chocolate mixture
- Bake at 350 degrees for 25-30 minutes or until set
- Let stand to cool, then cut into bars

92. Chocolate Drizzled Macaroons Recipe

Serving: 15 | Prep: | Cook: 20mins | Ready in:

Ingredients

- 14 oz. coconut
- 1/3 c. sugar
- 6 Tbsp. flour
- pinch of salt
- 4 egg whites
- 1/2 tsp. almond extract
- 1 c. semi-sweet chocolate chips, melted

Direction

- Mix coconut, sugar, flour and salt.
- Stir in egg whites and almond extract.
- Drop by spoonful onto greased & floured cookie sheet.
- Bake at 325 degrees for 15 min.

- Remove from cookie sheets and allow to cool completely on wire racks.
- Drizzle with melted chocolate.
- Refrigerate on wax paper-lined tray for at least 45 min.
- Makes 3 dozen

93. Chocolate Drizzlers Recipe

Serving: 80 | Prep: | Cook: 10mins | Ready in:

Ingredients

- 2 1/4 cups flour
- 1/3 cup cocoa powder
- 1/2 teaspoon baking soda
- 1/2 teaspoon baking powder
- 1/4 teaspoon salt
- 3/4 cup unsalted butter, softened
- 1 cup sugar
- 1 egg
- 4 ounces semi-sweet chocolate, melted and cooled
- 3 ounces semi-sweet chocolate, finely chopped
- 1 teaspoon vanilla extract
- 3 ounces white chocolate, finely chopped

Direction

- In a medium bowl, whisk together flour, cocoa, baking soda, baking powder, and salt. In another bowl, beat butter and sugar until creamy, about 2 minutes with an electric mixer. Beat in egg, 4 ounces of melted chocolate, and vanilla. Gradually beat in flour mixture until blended. Divide dough in half. Shape each half into a roll 2" in diameter. Wrap rolls in waxed paper and freeze for 4 hours or until very firm. Preheat oven to 350F. Line two baking sheets with foil and coat them with cooking spray.
- Cut dough into 1/4" slices. Arrange 1" apart on prepared baking sheets. Bake cookies 10 to 11 minutes. Cool on sheets for 1 minute then

transfer to wire racks to cool completely. Repeat process until all cookies are baked.
- To decorate the cookies, place the chopped milk chocolate in one small zip-lock baggie and the white chocolate in another. Microwave on high 1 minute or until chocolate is melted.
- Knead until smooth. Snip off a tiny corner of each bag and drizzle chocolate over cookie. Let cookies stand until chocolate is firm, about an hour.

94. Chocolate Frosted Coconut Cookies Recipe

Serving: 36 | Prep: | Cook: 10mins | Ready in:

Ingredients

- ----------- FOR 3 DOZEN cookies -----------
- 1/4 cup soft butter or margarine
- 3/4 cup sugar
- 2 eggs
- 1/2 cup sour cream
- 1/2 teaspoon vanilla
- 1/4 teaspoon baking soda
- 1/4 teaspoon baking powder
- 1/4 teaspoon salt
- 1 3/4 cups all-pupose flour
- 1 cup flaked coconut
- ---------- chocolate icing ----------
- 1 tablespoon butter or margarine
- 1 square (1oz) unsweetened chocoate
- 3 tblespoons cream or milk
- Dash salt
- 1/2 teaspoon vanilla 1 1/2 cups powdered sugar, not sifted, but free of lumps

Direction

- Preheat oven to 400.F
- Cream butter with sugar until blended. Add the eggs. Mix well.
- Stir in sour cream, vanilla, baking soda, baking powder and salt. Add flour and coconut. Mix until a stiff dough forms.

- Drop by rounded spoonfuls onto a lightly greased cookie sheet.
- Bake at 400.F for 8 to 10 minutes or until cookies are golden around the edges and firm to the touch.
- Frost while hot, with chocolate Icing.

95. Chocolate Hazelnut Krispy Squares Recipe

Serving: 16 | Prep: | Cook: 30mins | Ready in:

Ingredients

- 4 tablespoons (1/2 stick) butter
- 1 package (10 oz.) regular marshmallows or 4 cups miniature marshmallows
- 1 cup chocolate hazelnut spread (Nutella)
- 6 cups crispy style cereal   (Rice Krispies)
- 12 pieces of Ferrero Rocher fine hazelnut candies, buzzed for a pulse or two in a food processor, to break up, alternately, bash them with a rolling pin.

Direction

- Melt butter in a large saucepan over low heat.
- Add marshmallows and stir until completely melted.
- Remove from heat and stir in chocolate hazelnut spread until melted.
- Add cereal and bashed up candies.
- Stir with a wooden spoon or spatula until well coated.
- Try a little nonstick cooking spray on the spoon to keep it from sticking.
- Using a sheet of wax paper, evenly press mixture into a 13 x 9-inch pan coated with nonstick cooking spray.
- Cool completely.
- Cut into squares.

96. Chocolate Macadamia Cookies Recipe

Serving: 36 | Prep: | Cook: 8mins | Ready in:

Ingredients

- 1 pkg. choc. chip cookie mix
- 1/4 c. unsweetened cocoa powder
- 1/3 c. veg. oil
- 1 egg
- 3 tablespoons water
- 2/3 c. coarsely chopped macadamian nuts

Direction

- Preheat oven to 375.
- Combine cookie mix and cocoa in large bowl. Add oil, egg and water.
- Stir until thoroughly blended. Stir in macadamia nuts. Drop by rounded teaspoonful 2 inches apart onto an ungreased cookie sheet.
- Bake 8 to 10 minutes or until set. Cool 1 minute on cookie sheets.
- Remove to cooling racks. Cool completely.
- Makes 3 dozen cookies

97. Chocolate Mice Recipe

Serving: 12 | Prep: | Cook: 120mins | Ready in:

Ingredients

- 4 (1 ounce) squares semisweet chocolate
- 1/3 cup sour cream
- 1 cup chocolate cookie crumbs
- 1/3 cup chocolate cookie crumbs
- 1/3 cup confectioners sugar
- 24 silver dragees decorating candy
- 1/4 cup sliced almonds
- 12 (2inch) pieces long red vine licorice

Direction

- 1. Melt the chocolate, and combine with sour cream. Stir in 1 cup chocolate cookie crumbs. Cover and refrigerate until firm.
- 2. Roll by level tablespoonful into balls. Mold to a slight point at one end (the nose)
- 3. Roll dough in confectioners' sugar (for white mice), and in chocolate crumbs (for dark mice). On each mouse, place degrees in appropriate spot for eyes, almond slices for ears, and a licorice string for the tail.
- 4. Refrigerate for at least two hours, until firm.

98. Chocolate Mint Bars Recipe

Serving: 20 | Prep: | Cook: 23mins | Ready in:

Ingredients

- Bottom layer
- 1 cup all purpose flour(4 1/2 oz)
- 1/2 tsp salt
- 1 cup granulate sugar
- 1/2 cup egg substitute
- 1/4 cup butter,melted
- 2 tblsp water
- 1 tsp vanilla extract
- 2 large eggs,beaten
- 1 16 oz can chocolate syrup
- cooking spray
- mint LAYER
- 2 cups powdered sugar
- 1/4 cup butter,melted
- 2 tblsp fat free milk
- 1/2 tsp peppermint extract
- 2 drops green food coloring
- glaze
- 3/4 cup semi sweet chocolate chips
- 3 tblsp butter.

Direction

- Preheat oven to 350.
- To prepare bottom layer, lightly spoon flour into a measuring cup: level with a knife, combine flour and salt: stir with a whisk.

- Combine granulated sugar, egg substitute, 3/4cup melted butter, 2 tbsp. water, vanilla, eggs and chocolate syrup in a medium bowl; until smooth.
- Add flour mixture to chocolate mixture, stirring until blended.
- Pour batter into a 13 x9 baking pan coated with cooking spray.
- Bake at 350 for 23 min or until a wooden pick inserted comes out clean.
- Cool completely in pan on a wire rack.
- To prepare the mint layer:
- Combine powdered sugar, 1/4 cup melted butter, milk, peppermint extract, food coloring.
- In medium bowl; beat with a mixer until smooth.
- Spread mixture over cooled cake.
- To prepare the Glaze:
- Combine the chocolate chips and three tbsp. butter in a medium microwave safe bowl.
- Microwave high for 1 min or until melted, stirring after 30 sec.
- Let stand 2 min.
- Spread chocolate mixture evenly over top.
- Cover and refrigerate until ready to serve. Cut into 20 pieces.

99. Chocolate Mint Cookies Recipe

Serving: 36 | Prep: | Cook: 8mins | Ready in:

Ingredients

- Makes 3 dozens
- 3/4 cup butter
- 1 1/2 cups packed brown sugar
- 2 tablespoons water
- 2 cups semisweet chocolate chips
- 2 eggs
- 2 1/2 cups all-purpose flour
- 1 1/4 teaspoons baking soda
- 1/2 teaspoon salt

- 36 chocolate mint wafer candies (I used Andes mints)

Direction

- In a large pan over low heat, cook butter, sugar and water until butter is melted. Add chocolate chips and stir until partially melted. Remove from heat and continue to stir until chocolate is completely melted. Pour into a large bowl and let stand 10 minutes to cool off slightly.
- At high speed, beat in eggs, one at a time into chocolate mixture. Reduce speed to low and add dry ingredients, beating until blended. Chill dough about 1 hour.
- Preheat oven to 350 degrees F (175 degrees C). Roll dough into balls and place on ungreased cookie sheet about 2 inches apart. Bake 8-10 minutes. While cookies are baking unwrap mints and divide each in half. When cookies are brought out of the oven, put 1/2 mint on top of each cookie
- Let the mint sit for up to 5 minutes until melted, then spread the mint on top of the cookie. Eat and enjoy

100. Chocolate Oatmeal Bars Recipe

Serving: 0 | Prep: | Cook: 10mins | Ready in:

Ingredients

- 1/2 cup butter, softened
- 1/2 cup packed brown sugar
- 1 egg
- 1 tsp vanilla
- 1/2 cup flour
- 1/2 cup quick-cooking oats
- 1 cup (6 oz.) semisweet chocolate chips
- 1/2 cup chopped pecans

Direction

- In a large mixing bowl, cream the butter and sugar until light and fluffy.
- Beat in the egg and vanilla.
- Add the flour and oats.
- Mix well
- Pour into a lightly greased 11 x 7-inch baking pan
- Bake at 375 F for 15-20 minutes or until lightly browned.
- Cool on a wire rack for 3-5 minutes
- Sprinkle with the chips
- When melted, spread the chocolate over the bars.
- Top with the nuts
- Cool completely
- Cut into bars

101. Chocolate Peanut Butter Squares Recipe

Serving: 8 | Prep: | Cook: 10mins | Ready in:

Ingredients

- 1 1/2 c graham cracker crumbs
- 1 c icing sugar
- 1/2 c butter
- 3/4 c peanut butter
- 1 1/2 c chocolate chips
- 2 tsp shortening

Direction

- Combine graham crumbs and icing sugar.
- Melt butter and peanut butter then mix well with crumb mixture.
- Pat into a greased 8x8 baking pan.
- Melt chocolate chips and shortening then spread over crust.
- Refrigerate at least 2 hours then cut into squares. Yum!

102.   Chocolate Pecan Pumpkin Bars Recipe

Serving: 15 | Prep: | Cook: 30mins |Ready in:

Ingredients

- 1 cup white flour
- 1 cup whole wheat flour
- 3/4 cup granulated sugar
- 1 cup pecans very finely chopped
- 2 teaspoons baking powder
- 1 teaspoon ground cinnamon
- 1/2 teaspoon baking soda
- 1/2 teaspoon salt
- 4 large eggs beaten
- 1 teaspoon vanilla
- 15 ounce can pure pumpkin
- 1/2 cup canola oil
- 1/4 cup milk
- 1/2 cup miniature chocolate chips

Direction

- Preheat oven to 350.
- Lightly oil or coat a jelly roll pan with non-stick cooking spray and set aside.
- Whisk together flours, sugar, pecans, baking powder, cinnamon, baking soda and salt.
- In separate bowl combine eggs, pumpkin, canola oil, vanilla and milk.
- Add to dry mixture along with chocolate chips then stir to combine.
- Spread batter evenly in the prepared pan and bake for 25 minutes then cool on wire rack.

103.   Chocolate Pinwheels Recipe

Serving: 36 | Prep: | Cook: 20mins |Ready in:

Ingredients

- 1-1/4 cups butter
- 1-1/2 cups powdered sugar

- 1 egg
- 3 cups all purpose flour
- 1/4 teaspoon salt
- 1/4 cup cocoa

Direction

- Mix butter, sugar and egg then stir in flour and salt.
- Divide dough in half then stir cocoa into half the dough and refrigerate one hour.
- On floured pastry cloth roll plain dough into a rectangle.
- Roll chocolate dough the same size then place on top then roll out until 3/16" thick.
- Starting at the long edge roll dough into a log then wrap and chill for one hour or longer.
- Heat oven to 400 then slice dough into 1/8" slices.
- If dough crumbles while slicing let it warm a bit.
- Place 1" apart on ungreased baking sheets then bake 8 minutes until set but not brown.
- Remove from sheets immediately and cool on racks.

104.   Chocolate Pistachio Hazelnut Biscotti Recipe

Serving: 0 | Prep: | Cook: 35mins |Ready in:

Ingredients

- 2 cups all purpose flour
- 1/3 cup cocoa powder
- 1 1/2 cups granulated sugar
- 3 tablespoons baking powder
- 1 tablespoon espresso powder
- Pinch of salt
- 2 egg yolks
- 7 whole eggs
- 1 teaspoon vanilla
- 1/2 cup pistachio flour, finely grounded****
- 1 cup hazelnut meal, finely grounded

- ***** you can make your own by putting them in your food processor

Direction

- Mix all dry ingredients with Kitchen Aid paddle.
- Slowly add liquid ingredients until dough is formed.
- Roll into 10-inch logs.
- Line onto greased baking pan.
- Bake in preheated 325 degree oven for approximately 25 minutes, until slightly golden brown.
- When cooled, slice 1/2 inch thick and bake again, until crisp.
- Dip each half into hot, melted, white chocolate before serving.
- Yield: 4 1/2 12-ounce logs

105.   Chocolate Raspberry Cheesecake Bars Recipe

Serving: 12 | Prep: | Cook: 17mins | Ready in:

Ingredients

- Crust
- 1 Cup flour
- ¼ Cup powdered sugar
- ½ Cup margerine
- Filling
- ½ Cup raspberry jam
- 3 oz pkg cream cheese (softened)
- 2 Tbl milk
- 1 Cup (6oz) white chocolate chips
- glaze
- 2 oz (2 squares) semisweet baking chocolate
- 1 Tbl shortening

Direction

- Oven 375
- Blend flour and powdered sugar, cut in margarine until crumbly.

- Press mixture into 9 inch square pan
- Bake 15 to 17 minutes or until lightly browned
- Spread jam evenly over baked crust.
- In small bowl, beat cream cheese and milk until smooth.
- Add melted chips to cream cheese mixture; beat until smooth.
- Drop cream cheese mixture by spoonfuls onto jam, spread evenly with a light hand
- Chill until set
- In small saucepan over low heat melt chocolate with shortening, stirring constantly.
- Spread over white chocolate layer. Chill completely, cut into bars.
- Cover and refrigerate

106.   Chow Mein Candy Recipe

Serving: 10 | Prep: | Cook: 5mins | Ready in:

Ingredients

- 1 package chocolate chips
- 1 cup butterscotch chips
- 1 can chow mein noodles
- 1 cup cashew nuts, chopped

Direction

- Melt chocolate and butterscotch chips in top of double boiler.
- Remove from heat; stir in chow mein noodles and cashew nuts.
- Drop by spoonful onto waxed paper.
- Let cool.

107.   Christmas Window Biscuits Recipe

Serving: 0 | Prep: | Cook: 45mins | Ready in:

Ingredients

- 125g butter (cubed and at room temperature)
- 125g golden caster sugar
- 225g plain flour, plus extra for dusting
- 1/2 teaspoon vanilla extract
- 2 table spoons of milk
- 1 packet of colourful boiled sweets

Direction

- Preheat the oven to 180°C / Gas Mark 4 / Fan 160°C
- Line 2 baking sheets with greaseproof paper
- Put the butter and sugar into a large mixing bowl and whisk together until pale and fluffy
- Sift the flour into the mixture
- Add the milk
- Use your hands to mix everything together until you have a ball of dough
- Sprinkle a clean work surface with flour and place the dough in the center
- Lightly flour your rolling pin and roll the dough out until it's about 6mm thick
- Cut out your biscuits using large Christmas shaped cutters or a knife (ask an adult for help)
- Transfer each biscuit to the baking sheet, leaving plenty of space between each one
- Next carefully cut out the shapes for the window, using smaller cutters or a knife
- Place a boiled sweet into each window - if they are large sweets you can break them up by bashing them once or twice with a rolling pin whilst they are still in their wrappers
- Using a fat straw cut out a small hole for the ribbon
- Bake in the oven for 12 - 15 minutes or until they are a light golden brown and the sweets have melted
- Leave the biscuits to cool completely on the baking sheets as the sweets are very hot and need to set. When completely cool transfer to a wire rack
- Thread ribbon through each hole and they are ready to decorate your Christmas tree

108. Chunky Peanut Butter Triangles Recipe

Serving: 42 | Prep: | Cook: 18mins | Ready in:

Ingredients

- 1 1/2 cups all-purpose flour
- 1/2 teaspoon baking soda
- 3/4 cup creamy peanut butter
- 1/2 cup light butter softened
- 1/3 cup packed Splenda brown sugar blend
- 1/4 cup splenda suga blend for baking
- 1 large egg
- 1 teaspoon vanilla extract
- 1 3/4 cups nestle toll house semi sweet chocolate chunks

Direction

- Preheat oven to 350F
- COMBINE flour and baking soda in small bowl
- Beat peanut butter splenda brown sugar blend and splenda sugar blend for baking I large mixer bowl until creamy
- Beat in egg and vanilla extract
- Gradually beat in flour mixture
- Stir in chunks
- Press into ungreased 13x9-inch baking pan distributing chunks evenly
- Bake for 18 to minutes or until center is set. Cool completely in pan on wire rack. Cut into triangles

109. Cinnamon Cream Cheese Squares Recipe

Serving: 10 | Prep: | Cook: 30mins | Ready in:

Ingredients

- 2 8oz tubes refrigerated crescent rolls

- 16 oz cream cheese (softened)
- 1 1/2 cups granulated sugar - divided
- 3 tbls butter or margarine, melted
- 1 tsp. ground cinnamon
- 1 tsp. vanilla extract

Direction

- Preheat oven to 350°F
- Unroll 1 tube of crescent rolls
- Place in lightly greased 13x9 baking pan, seal seams and set aside
- In mixing bowl, beat cream cheese, 1 cup of sugar and vanilla extract until smooth.
- Spread over dough
- Unroll 2nd crescent rolls and place over cream cheese mix, stretching to fit.
- Brush butter on top
- Combine cinnamon and remaining sugar and sprinkle on top
- Bake for 30 minutes

110. Coco Nutty Tropical Treat Bars Recipe

Serving: 32 | Prep: | Cook: 25mins | Ready in:

Ingredients

- 2 cups graham cracker crumbs
- 1/4 cup confectioners' sugar
- 1 stick (8 tablespoons) butter, melted
- 1 can (14 ounces) sweetened condensed milk
- 1 can (8 ounces) crushed pineapple in juice, drained and excess
- moisture squeezed out
- 1 can (7 ounces) sweetened shredded coconut
- 1/2 cup coarsely chopped almonds, pecans or macadamia nuts
- 1 1/2 cups white chocolate chips

Direction

- Heat oven to 375°F. Grease a 9x13-inch baking pan.

- Mix graham cracker crumbs and confectioners' sugar. Stir in butter until evenly moistened. Press crumb mixture firmly into bottom of pan. Bake until edges are golden brown, 10 to 12 minutes.
- Meanwhile stir sweetened condensed milk, pineapple, coconut and almonds until blended. Pour into baked crust and spread almost to edges.
- Bake until just set, 10 to 15 minutes. Remove from oven and sprinkle with white chocolate chips. Let stand until chocolate softens, 3 to 4 minutes, then carefully spread chocolate over surface.
- Cool completely. Cut into 32 bars.

111. Cocoa Sticks Recipe

Serving: 12 | Prep: | Cook: 5mins | Ready in:

Ingredients

- 6 tablespoonfuls butter
- 3/4 cup granulated sugar
- 1 egg
- 1 tablespoon milk
- 1 teaspoon vanilla
- 5 teaspoonfuls cocoa
- 1/8 teaspoon baking powder
- 1-1/2 cups sifted pastry flour

Direction

- Cream butter until soft then add sugar gradually and beat well.
- Add egg, milk and vanilla then mix thoroughly.
- Sift cocoa, baking powder and a pinch of salt with one-half cup of the flour.
- Stir this into the mixture first then use the remainder of the flour to make a firm dough.
- Set on the ice to harden then sprinkle board with cocoa and a little sugar.
- Use small pieces of the dough at a time and toss it over the board to prevent sticking.

- Roll out thin then cut in strips about 1/2" wide and 3" long.
- Place closely in pan and bake in moderately hot oven three or four minutes.

112. Coconut Bars Recipe

Serving: 48 | Prep: | Cook: |Ready in:

Ingredients

- 1/2 cup milk
- 1/2 cup butter
- 1 cup brown sugar
- 2 cups oatmeal
- 1 cup coconut
- 1 tsp vanilla
- 1 tsp salt

Direction

- Mix first 3 ingredients and bring to a boil until it bubbles, then remove from heat. Mix in the remaining ingredients.
- Press into an 8"x8" pan and cool until firm. Cut into bars approx. 1"x1" pieces.
- Heat 8 oz. of chocolate chips. Dip bars into chocolate and cool. The original recipe as written by my mother included 1/2 bar of paraffin wax with the chocolate chips - I make it without the paraffin - I think the only change is the firmness of the chocolate.

113. Coconut Chip Cookies Recipe

Serving: 41 | Prep: | Cook: 10mins |Ready in:

Ingredients

- 1 package (18 1/4 ounce) white cake mix
- 2 eggs
- 1/2 cup vegetable oil

- 1 cup flaked coconut
- 1/2 cp semisweet chocolate chips
- 1/4 cup chopped macadamia nuts or almonds

Direction

- In a mixing bowl, beat cake mix, eggs and oil (batter will be very stiff). Stir in coconut, chips, and nuts. Roll into 1 inch balls. Place on lightly greased baking sheets. Bake at 350 degrees for 10 minutes or until a slight indentation remains when lightly touched. Cool for 2 minutes remove to a wire rack to cool completely.

114. Coconut Dream Squares Recipe

Serving: 36 | Prep: | Cook: 25mins |Ready in:

Ingredients

- 1-1/4 cup sifted cake flour
- 1-1/4 cup firmly packed brown sugar
- 1/3 cup soft butter
- 2 eggs
- 1/2 teaspoon baking powder
- 1 teaspoon vanilla
- 1 cup chopped walnuts
- 1-1/3 cup flaked coconut

Direction

- Combine 1 cup of the flour and 1/4 cup of the sugar.
- Add butter and blend well then press firmly in ungreased square pan.
- Bake 15 minutes at 350.
- Meanwhile beat eggs until light.
- Add 1 cup sugar gradually beating constantly until fluffy.
- Sift 1/4 cup flour and baking powder then fold into egg mixture.
- Add vanilla, nuts and coconut then mix well.

- Spread over baked mixture in pan and bake 25 minutes.
- Cool and cut into squares.

115. Coconut Macaroons Recipe

Serving: 212 | Prep: | Cook: 15mins | Ready in:

Ingredients

- 3 Cups shredded coconut
- 1 1/2 tbps cornstarch
- 3/4 cup sugar
- 3 egg whites
- 1/2 tsp vanillia
- 4 ounces of sweet chocolete pieces

Direction

- Heat oven to 350; mix coconut, cornstarch, sugar, egg whites and vanilla in a heat proof bowl.
- Set bowl over a pot of boiling water (or use a double boiler)
- Heat stirring until mixture thickens (4) min then set aside.
- Spoon out mixture (about a tablespoon) and place on ungreased cooking sheet.
- Bake for 10-15 min. until golden brown (but still soft)
- Melt chocolate then dip macaroon bottoms letting chocolate drip off
- Place on wax paper until they are set.

116. Coffee Squares Recipe

Serving: 15 | Prep: | Cook: 40mins | Ready in:

Ingredients

- 2 eggs
- 2 2/3 cup light brown sugar

- 1 cup oil
- 1 cup warm strong coffee
- 1 teaspoon salt
- 1 teaspoon baking soda
- 3 cups flour
- 1 cup chopped walnuts
- 1- 12 ounce package semi-sweet chocolate chips

Direction

- Preheat oven to 350 degrees.
- Beat eggs in a large bowl, add sugar and oil and mix well.
- Stir in coffee, flour, baking soda and salt.
- Mix thoroughly and pour into greased 9 x 13 pan.
- Top with chocolate chips and walnuts.
- Bake 35-40 minutes.

117. Colorful MampM Cookies Recipe

Serving: 36 | Prep: | Cook: 11mins | Ready in:

Ingredients

- 1 cup Crisco shortening
- 1 cup packed light brown sugar
- 1/2 cup sugar
- 2 large eggs
- 1 teaspoon vanilla
- 2 1/4 cups flour
- 1 teaspoon salt
- 1 teaspoon baking soda
- 1 1/2 cups M&M's plain chocolate candy

Direction

- 1) Cream together shortening and sugars until light and fluffy.
- 2) Add eggs and vanilla and beat until combined.
- 3) Add combined flour, salt, and baking soda and mix until well combined.

- 4) Stir in 1/2 cup M&Ms.
- 5) Drop by Tbsp. onto ungreased cookie sheet.
- 6) Press 2-3 M&Ms onto top of each cookie.
- 7) Bake in 375°F for 10-12 minutes.

118. Cookie Fruit Cobbler Recipe

Serving: 12 | Prep: | Cook: 24mins | Ready in:

Ingredients

- * 2 cans (21 oz. each) cherry, peach, blueberry or apple pie filling
- * 1 package (18-oz.) NESTLÉ TOLL HOUSE Refrigerated chocolate chip Cookie Bar Dough
- * 1 cup quick or old-fashioned oats

Direction

- PREHEAT oven to 375° F. Grease 13 x 9-inch baking pan.
- SPOON pie filling into pan.
- CRUMBLE cookie dough into medium bowl. Add oats; mix well. Sprinkle over filling.
- BAKE for 24 to 28 minutes or until top is deep golden brown. Serve warm or at room temperature.

119. Copycat Mrs Fields Peanut Butter Cookies Recipe

Serving: 30 | Prep: | Cook: 60mins | Ready in:

Ingredients

- 1/4   tsp. salt
- 1/2   tsp. baking soda
- 2   cups flour
- 2   tsp. vanilla
- 1   cup creamy peanut butter
- 3   eggs

- 1   cup softened butter
- 1 1/4 cup sugar
- 1 1/4 cup dark brown sugar

Direction

- Preheat oven to 300*
- In a medium sized bowl, combine the flour, baking soda, and salt. Mix together with a wire whisk
- In a large bowl, blend the sugars with an electric mixer at medium speed.
- Add butter and mix until it forms a paste.
- Next, add the eggs, peanut butter, and vanilla.
- Mix at medium speed until the batter becomes light and fluffy.
- Add the flour mixture and change the mixer to low speed. Continue until just mixed.
- Drop by tablespoons onto an ungreased cookie sheet, 1 1/2" apart.
- With a fork, gently press a crisscross pattern on top of each cookie.
- Bake for 10-20 minutes until cookies are slightly brown along the edges.
- Transfer cookies to a wire rack to cool.

120. Cranberry Coconut Chews Recipe

Serving: 0 | Prep: | Cook: 1hours | Ready in:

Ingredients

- 3 sticks of unsalted butter, room temperature
- 2 cups sugar
- 1 tablespoon grated orange peel
- 2 teaspoons pure vanilla extract
- 1 large egg
- 3-1/4 cups all-purpose flour
- 1 teaspoon baking powder
- 1/4 teaspoon salt
- 1-1/2 cups dried cranberries
- 1-1/2 cups sweetened flaked dried coconut

Direction

- In large bowl, with mixer on medium speed, place butter, sugar, orange peel and vanilla
- Beat until smooth
- Beat in egg until well blended
- In medium bowl, mix flour, baking powder, salt
- Add to butter mixture, stirring to mix
- Beat on low speed until dough comes together (about 5 minutes)
- Mix in cranberries and coconut
- Shape dough into 1-inch balls, placing 2 inches apart on buttered cookie sheet (may use cookie scoop)
- Bake in a 350 degree oven until cookies begin to brown slightly, about 11 minutes.....15 minutes for a crisper cookie
- Cool baked cookies on sheet for 5 minutes, then transfer to racks to cool completely

121.   Cream Cheese Balls Recipe

Serving: 12 | Prep: | Cook: | Ready in:

Ingredients

- 2-1/2 cups powdered sugar sifted
- 3 ounces cream cheese softened
- 1/4 teaspoon vanilla
- 1/8 teaspoon salt
- 7 ounces shredded coconut

Direction

- In mixer gradually add sugar to softened cream cheese mixing until well blended.
- Mix in vanilla and salt then shape batter into bite size balls and roll in shredded coconut.
- Place on a tray or in a plastic or glass container so that they are not touching each other.
- Refrigerate overnight before serving.

122.   Cream Cheese Cookies Recipe

Serving: 0 | Prep: | Cook: 45mins | Ready in:

Ingredients

- 2 8-oz pkg. cream cheese, softened
- 2 c. granulated sugar
- 3 c. all-purpose flour
- 1 T. white vinegar
- 2 tsp. baking soda
- 2 c. chopped walnuts (we coarsely grind ours)
- Additional sugar for rolling cookies

Direction

- Preheat oven to 325 degrees F.
- Cream sugar and cream cheese until light and fluffy. Beat in vinegar.
- In a separate bowl, combine flour, soda and walnuts.
- Gradually add flour mixture to sugar and cream cheese mixture. Chill cookie dough for about an hour.
- Drop by teaspoonful (I use a small cookie scoop) into a bowl of sugar and roll to coat. Place on baking sheet about 1" apart and flatten slightly. I use the bottom of a glass. If the balls haven't been rolled in sugar, dip glass in sugar to prevent sticking.
- Put cookie sheet in preheated oven for 18 minutes. Remove from oven and allow to cool for a couple of minutes before removing from sheet. Once removed from sheet, cool completely and store in an airtight container. (We use a zip-lock bag.)
- NOTES:
- 1. This dough is very sticky due to using cream cheese instead of butter. Rolling them in sugar makes the balls much easier to handle.
- 2. These cookies do not spread. If left in a mound, they will come out as a mound. Those are good too, but we like them better flattened because it gives more surface for the crispy.

123.   Cream Cheese Delights Recipe

Serving: 24 | Prep: | Cook: 15mins | Ready in:

Ingredients

- 1/2 cup butter-flavored shortening
- 1 pkg. (3 oz.) cream cheese, softened
- 1/2 cup sugar
- 1 egg yolk
- 1 tsp vanilla
- 1 cup flour
- 1 tsp salt
- Halved maraschino cherries or candied cherries

Direction

- In a small bowl, cream the shortening, cream cheese, and sugar until light and fluffy.
- Beat in the egg yolk and vanilla.
- Combine the flour and salt.
- Gradually add to the creamed mixture.
- Mix well.
- Drop by teaspoonful 2 inches apart onto greased baking sheets.
- Top each with a cherry half.
- Bake at 350°F for 12-15 minutes or until lightly browned.
- Cool for 1 minute before removing to wire racks.

124.   Crispy Chocolate Bars Recipe

Serving: 32 | Prep: | Cook: 5mins | Ready in:

Ingredients

- 1 Pkge semi sweet chocolaete morsels
- 1 cup butterscotch morsels
- 1/2 cup peanut butter

- 5 cups cornflakes - I bet rice crispys would work too =)

Direction

- In 3 quart saucepan, combine chocolate morsels, butterscotch morsels and peanut butter. Stir over low heat till melted and smooth.
- Remove from heat and stir in the cornflakes till evenly coated
- Using a buttered spatula or wax paper press mixture evenly into a 9x9x2 inch pan coated with cooking spray. Let cool completely
- Cut into squares, store in airtight container.
- Even quicker - Morsels can be melted in the microwave!

125.   Crunchy Choc Oat No Bakes Recipe

Serving: 15 | Prep: | Cook: 10mins | Ready in:

Ingredients

- ½ cup raw sugar
- ¼ cup white sugar
- ¼ cup butter
- ¼ cup milk
- ¼ cup peanut paste
- 1 cup oats
- 2 Tbsp cocoa
- handful each: sultanas, cornflakes, rice bubbles

Direction

- - Combine sugars, butter and milk in a saucepan. Heat until it's all melted together, then boil, stirring for about 2 minutes.
- - Remove from heat. Stir in peanut paste and vanilla.
- - In a large bowl, have ready the remaining ingredients.
- - Pour saucepan contents onto dry ingredients and mix well.

- - Drop Tablespoonful of mixture onto a lined tray. Leave until set.

126. Currant Cookies Recipe

Serving: 60 | Prep: | Cook: 10mins | Ready in:

Ingredients

- 4 cups flour
- 1 1/2 cups granulated sugar
- 1 tbsp. baking powder
- 3/4 tsp. ground nutmeg
- 1/2 tsp. salt
- 1 cup vegetable shortening
- 1/4 cup milk
- 3 large eggs, beaten
- 1 cup dried currants

Direction

- In large bowl, combine flour, granulated sugar, baking powder, nutmeg and salt; mix well. Cut in shortening with a pastry blender until crumbly.
- Add enough milk to beaten eggs to measure 1 cup. Stir into flour mixture. Stir in currants. Cover; chill for 1 hour.
- Preheat griddle to 350°F. Lightly oil griddle.
- On lightly floured surface, roll dough out to 1/4 inch thick. Cut with cookie cutter.
- Cook on griddle 3 minutes per side or until golden.

127. DOUBLE DELICIOUS COOKIE BARS Recipe

Serving: 18 | Prep: | Cook: 30mins | Ready in:

Ingredients

- 1 1/2 C. graham cracker crumbs
- 1/2 C. (1 stick) butter or margarine
- 1 (14-oz.) can sweetened condensed milk
- 1 C. (6 oz) semi-sweet chocolate chips
- 1 C. (6 oz.) peanut butter-flavored chips

Direction

- Preheat oven to 350°F (325°F for glass dish).
- In small bowl, combine graham cracker crumbs and butter; mix well. Press crumb mixture firmly on bottom of 13X9-inch baking pan.
- Pour Sweetened Condensed Milk evenly over crumb mixture.
- Layer evenly with remaining ingredients; press down firmly with fork.
- Bake 25 to 30 minutes or until lightly browned.
- Cool.
- Cut into bars.
- Store leftovers covered at room temperature.

128. Danish Pastry Apple Bars Recipe

Serving: 12 | Prep: | Cook: 60mins | Ready in:

Ingredients

- 2 1/2 Cups all-purpose flour
- 1 Tsp.salt
- 1 Cup shortening
- 1 ,egg yolk
- 1/2 cup milk
- 10 apples,peeled,cored and thinly sliced
- 1/2 cup light brown sugar
- 1/4 cup white sugar
- 1/2 Tsp.cinnamon
- 1/4 Tsp.nutmeg
- 1 egg white

Direction

- Preheat oven to 375 F (190 C)
- In large bowl, combine flour and salt. Cut in shortening until mixture resembles coarse crumbs. Beat egg yolk in measuring cup and

add enough milk to make 2/3 cup total liquid. Stir into flour mixture until all flour is damp. Divide the dough in half. On floured surface, roll half the dough into a rectangle and fit into a 9 X 13 pan.

- In large bowl, combine apples, sugars, cinnamon and nutmeg. Put apple mixture in pan. Roll out remaining dough and place over apples. Seal edges and cut slits in top dough. Beat egg white till frothy and brush on crust.
- Bake in preheated oven for 50 minutes, or until golden brown.

129. Dark Chocolate And Mint Whoopie Pies Recipe

Serving: 20 | Prep: | Cook: 11mins | Ready in:

Ingredients

- cookiE
- 3/4 cup (1 1/2 sticks) unsalted butter, room temperature
- 3/4 cup dark brown sugar
- 2 eggs
- 3 cups flour
- 3/4 cup unsweetened cocoa powder
- 2 teasp. baking soda
- 1 teasp. salt
- 1 1/2 cups low-fat buttermilk
- 1 1/2 teasp. vanilla
- 1/2 teasp. instant coffee
- ....
- FILLING
- 3/4 cup (1 1/2 sticks) unsalted butter, room temperature
- 1 teasp. vanilla
- 1/2 teasp. mint extract or 1 TBSP. finely chopped fresh mint
- 2 3/4 cups powdered sugar, sifted
- 3 cups marshmallow fluff
- optional.... couple of drops of green food coloring.

Direction

- COOKIES
- In large mixing bowl with mixer set on medium speed. Mix butter and sugar until well blended....about 3 minutes
- Add eggs, one at a time mixing until smooth after each
- Mix in vanilla
- In another bowl... stir together flour, cocoa powder, baking soda, and salt
- In a 2-cup liquid measuring cup stir together buttermilk and instant coffee unto the coffee has dissolved... this make take a minute or two ...set aside
- Add 1/2 the flour mixture to butter mixture and mix on medium speed until combined and smooth
- Add 1/2 buttermilk beat on medium speed until smooth and slightly fluffy in texture
- Repeat with the remaining flour and then the buttermilk
- Batter will be thick and slightly springy when done
- Spray 2 baking sheet with cooking spray
- Drop 2 tablespoons of batter onto the baking sheets
- Leave 2-inches between to allow for spreading
- Bake in a preheated 350' F oven for 11 - 13 minutes... until they are puffed and set but still soft when touched lightly with fingertips
- Let cakes cool 3 minutes on the baking sheets then transfer to wire rack to finish cooling ... about 15 - 20 minutes
- ....
- FILLING
- Large bowl ... sift powdered sugar
- Set aside
- In large mixer bowl ...mixer on medium... butter, vanilla and mint until creamy
- Add 1/2 the powdered sugar
- Mix on low speed first to combine then on high until smooth
- Repeat with remaining powdered sugar.
- Add marshmallow cream
- Mix on medium-high until filling is light and fluffy, about 3 to 4 minutes

- ....
- ASSEMBLE....
- Spoon filling onto flat side of 1/2 the cakes
- Dividing evenly between them
- Top with remaining cakes flat side against the filling
- Round sides of the filling up. So it looks nice
- Serve immediately or wrap each one individually in plastic wrap
- Store room temperature for up to 2 days or in the freezer

130. Date Coffee Squares Recipe

Serving: 12 | Prep: | Cook: 30mins | Ready in:

Ingredients

- 1 cup dates
- 1 cup hot coffee
- 1 cup butter
- 1 cup granulated sugar
- 2 eggs
- 1-3/4 cups flour
- 1 tablespoon cocoa
- 1 teaspoon baking soda
- 12 ounce bag chocolate chips
- 1 cup chopped pecans

Direction

- In blender combine dates and hot coffee then blend and cool.
- Cream butter, sugar and eggs.
- Add flour, cocoa and baking soda alternately with date mixture.
- Mix in bag of chips and nuts then bake in greased pan at 350 for 30 minutes.

131. Date Squares Recipe

Serving: 24 | Prep: | Cook: 20mins | Ready in:

Ingredients

- Base
- 1 1/2 cups cake flour
- 1 1/2 cups rolled oats
- 1 cup packed brown sugar
- 1/2 tsp baking soda
- 1/4 tsp salt
- 3/4 cups butter or margarine
- date Paste
- 1 pound dried dates
- 1/3 cup brown sugar (optional as dates are very sweet)
- 1/2 cup orange juice
- 1/2 cup water
- 1/2 tsp vanilla extract

Direction

- Pre-heat oven to 350 f.
- Place dates in a pot with sugar, orange juice and water over medium heat
- Cook and mash with a fork or potato masher until you get a paste
- Add vanilla and set aside to cool
- Mix all of the dry ingredients together and add butter or margarine
- With your hand combine everything until you get a crumbly mixture
- Split mixture in half and place in a 9x9 inch greased pan
- Press down slightly to create a crust
- Carefully place the date paste on top of the crust
- Loosely place the rest of the "crumbs" on top of the date paste but DO NOT press down on it to create a crust
- Place in the oven for 20 mins
- Let it cool before cutting
- Enjoy!

132. Delightful Cream Cheese Bars Recipe

Serving: 12 | Prep: | Cook: 20mins | Ready in:

Ingredients

- 1 stick margarine
- 1 cup flour
- 1 cup finely chopped pecans
- 8 ounces cream cheese softened
- 1 cup powdered sugar
- 8 ounces frozen whipped topping thawed
- 1 large chocolate instant pudding

Direction

- In a rectangular baking dish mix margarine, flour and 3/4 cup pecans.
- Press down in bottom to make crust then bake at 400° for 20 minutes then cool completely.
- Mix cream cheese, powdered sugar and whipping topping in bowl then spread on cooled crust.
- Mix pudding as directed for pie then spread on top of cream cheese layer.
- Top with remaining whipped topping and sprinkle with remaining nuts.
- Let chill at least one hour before serving.

133. Devils Food Cookies Recipe

Serving: 24 | Prep: | Cook: 12mins | Ready in:

Ingredients

- 1 1/2 cups sugar
- 1 1/4 cups shortening
- 1/2 cup cocoa
- 3 eggs
- 2 tsp baking soda
- 1 tsp salt
- 2 1/4 cups flour

Direction

- Mix all ingredients (except flour) until fluffy
- Add flour and mix thoroughly
- Make balls of dough about 1 inch and roll in sugar
- Flatten cookies slightly
- Bake at 350 for 12 min + -
- Cool on wire rack
- Enjoy

134. Diamond Crumble Bars Recipe

Serving: 36 | Prep: | Cook: 25mins | Ready in:

Ingredients

- • 1 cup (2 sticks) butter, softened
- • 2 1/4 cups all-purpose flour
- • 1/2 cup granulated sugar
- • 1/4 teaspoon salt
- • 2 cups (12-oz. pkg.) NESTLÉ® TOLL HOUSE® Semi-sweet chocolate Morsels, divided
- • 1 can (14 oz.) NESTLÉ® CARNATION® sweetened condensed milk
- • 1 teaspoon vanilla extract
- • 1 cup chopped pecans, toasted

Direction

- PREHEAT oven to 350° F. Grease 13 x 9-inch baking pan.
- BEAT butter in large mixer bowl on medium speed for 30 seconds. Beat in flour, sugar and salt on low speed until crumbly. Press 2 cups of mixture onto bottom of prepared pan. Bake for 12 to 14 minutes or until lightly browned on edges.
- COMBINE 1 1/2 cups of morsels and sweetened condensed milk in small saucepan over medium-low heat. Heat until morsels are melted, stirring constantly. Remove from heat; stir in vanilla extract. Pour evenly over hot

crust. Add remaining morsels and chopped pecans to the reserved crust mixture; sprinkle over the chocolate layer.

- BAKE for 25 to 30 minutes or until center is set. Cool in pan on wire rack. Cut into diamond-shaped pieces.
- The smooth chocolate filling is a marvellous contrast to the crumb layers and crunchy chocolate pecan topping. Carrie Singh of Naples, FL developed this recipe

---

135.   Dog Biscuits Recipe

Serving: 12 | Prep: | Cook: 45mins |Ready in:

Ingredients

- 1 lb turkey (bones removed)
- 1 lb pork
- 4 slices of bacon
- 2 eggs, beaten
- 2 cups all-purpose flour
- 1 cup cornmeal

Direction

- Shred the turkey, pork, bacon and eggs in your food processor & set aside.
- In a mixing bowl, combine the turkey/pork/bacon/egg mixture with your hands & mix well.
- You can mix everything in a food processor if you have one that is big enough.
- (Skip this step if you mixed all of the ingredients in a food processor.)
- Knead dough in a large bowl until the dough ball isn't sticky anymore. It takes about 2 minutes.
- Lightly grease a cookie sheet (9"x15")
- Use a rolling pin to roll out dough in the cookie sheet until it's 1/4 to 1/2 inch thick.
- Use a pizza cutter to slice the dough into 1-inch squares
- Bake for 1 hour in oven preheated to 375° F

- If you decide to use meat in this recipe that is already cooked, cut the cooking time down to 45 minutes.
- Cool before giving any to your dog. Store the rest in the refrigerator.

---

136.   Double Delicious Cookie Bars Recipe

Serving: 24 | Prep: | Cook: 25mins |Ready in:

Ingredients

- Ingredients:
- 1/2 cup (1 stick) butter or margarine
- 1-1/2 cups graham cracker crumbs
- 1 can (14 oz.) sweetened condensed milk (not evaporated milk)
- 2 cups (12-oz. pkg.) HERSHEY'S SPECIAL dark chocolate chips or HERSHEY'S semi-sweet chocolate chips
- 1 cup REESE'S peanut butter chips
- 1 cup HERSHEY'S SPECIAL dark chocolate chips or HERSHEY'S semi-sweet chocolate chips
- 1-1/2 teaspoons shortening(do not use butter, margarine, spread or oil)

Direction

- Directions:
- Heat oven to 350°F. (325°F. for glass dish).
- Melt butter in oven in 13x9x2-inch baking pan. Sprinkle graham cracker crumbs over butter; pour sweetened condensed milk evenly over crumbs. Top with 2 cups chocolate chips and peanut butter chips; press down firmly.
- Bake 25 to 30 minutes or until lightly browned. Cool completely in pan on wire rack. Place 1 cup chocolate chips and shortening in small microwave-safe bowl. Microwave at MEDIUM (50%) 1 to 1-1/2 minutes or until smooth when stirred. Drizzle over top of bars. When drizzle is firm, cut into bars. Store loosely covered at room temperature. 24 to 36 bars.

137.   Drömkakor Recipe

Serving: 0 | Prep: | Cook: 25mins | Ready in:

Ingredients

- 1 2/3 cake flour
- 1 teaspoon baking soda
- 1 stick unsalted butter, softened
- 1 1/4 cups sugar
- 1 tablespoon vanilla sugar
- 1/8 tsp almond extract
- 1/3 cup corn oil

Direction

- Preheat oven to 300 degrees. In a small bowl, whisk flour and baking soda and set aside. In a large bowl, beat butter and sugars until light and fluffy. Add oil and extracts and mix until smooth. Add dry ingredients and stir until just combined. Roll dough into 1 inch balls (about 1 teaspoonful) and place about 2 inches apart on parchment paper lined baking sheets.
- Bake for 20 minutes or until cookies are just set and crack on the top. Cool on a wire rack.
- Makes about 3 dozen cookies

138.   Dulce De Leche Cream Cheese Cookies Easy Recipe

Serving: 4 | Prep: | Cook: | Ready in:

Ingredients

- Goya Dulce de Leche Maria cookies (or any other sweet cracker/cookie you may have)
- cream cheese
- caramel syrup/sauce (the thicker and richer the better)

Direction

- Take cracker/cookie
- Smear on cream cheese
- Top with caramel
- Eat
- Yes! It is that easy!
- If you want to get a little fancy, chop up and sprinkle on some glazed pecans.

139.   Dump Truck Bars Recipe

Serving: 18 | Prep: | Cook: 8mins | Ready in:

Ingredients

- 2 - Cups confectioners sugar
- 1 - 13 oz can evaporated milk
- 1 - 6 oz package chocolate chips
- 1/2 Cup butter
- 1 - 15 oz. package (about 42) Oreo cookies, crushed
- 1/2 Cup melted butter.
- 1 tsp. vanilla extract
- 1 1/2 Cups Spanish peanuts
- 1/2 Gallon vanilla ice cream, softened

Direction

- Combine confectioners' sugar, evaporated milk, chocolate chips and 1/2 cup butter in saucepan.
- Boil for 8 minutes, stirring constantly. Add vanilla and cool.
- Combine crushed cookies with 1/2 melted butter.
- Pat into greased 9x13 " baking dish and freeze until firm.
- Sprinkle with Spanish peanuts over cookie crust.
- Spread softened ice cream over peanuts and cover with cooled chocolate sauce.
- Freeze until ready to serve. Slice into bars.

140. Dutch Butterscotch Apple Squares Recipe

Serving: 12 | Prep: | Cook: 30mins |Ready in:

Ingredients

- 1/4 cup margarine
- 1-1/2 cups graham cracker crumbs
- 1-1/4 cups peeled chopped apples
- 1 (6 oz.) package butterscotch chips
- 1 (14 oz.) can sweetened condensed milk
- 1 (3-1/2 oz.) can flaked coconut
- 1 cup chopped nuts

Direction

- Preheat oven to 350 degrees.
- In 13x9-inch baking pan, melt margarine in oven.
- Sprinkle graham cracker crumbs evenly over margarine; top with apples.
- In heavy sauce pan, over medium heat, melt butterscotch chips with sweetened condensed milk.
- Pour butterscotch mixture evenly over apples.
- Top with coconut and nuts; press down firmly.
- Bake 25 to 30 minutes or until lightly browned. Cool. Chill thoroughly

141. Easy Chocolate Chip Cookie Cream Cheese Cake Recipe

Serving: 24 | Prep: | Cook: 30mins |Ready in:

Ingredients

- 2-16 ounce packages refrigerated chocolate chip cookie dough
- 2-8 ounce packages Philadelphia cream cheese, softened
- 2 eggs
- 1 cup sugar
- 1-1/2 teaspoons vanilla

Direction

- Place cookie dough packages in the freezer for about 30 minutes
- This makes it easier to slice
- Grease and flour a 9 X 13 inch baking dish or pan
- Remove one package of cookie dough from the freezer
- Slice into 1/4 inch thick slices
- Place the slices in the bottom of the baking dish or pan
- It's okay if they overlap
- In bowl, mix cream cheese, eggs, sugar and vanilla together
- Blend well
- Spread over the layer of cookie dough in the dish or pan
- Remove the other package of dough from the freezer
- Slice into 1/4 inch thick slices
- Place slices on top of the cream cheese mixture
- Bake 30-35 minutes in a 350 degree oven
- Can be cut to serve 24

142. Easy Fudge Cookis Recipe

Serving: 42 | Prep: | Cook: 10mins |Ready in:

Ingredients

- 1 18 1/4 oz. Betty Crocker Super Moist devil's food cake mix
- 1/2 cup vegetable oil
- 2 large eggs
- confectioner's sugar for rolling

Direction

- Preheat oven to 350.
- Stir dry cake mix, oil and eggs in a large bowl, by hand, until dough forms.

- Dust hands with confectioner's sugar and form dough into 1 " balls.
- Roll balls in confectioners' sugar and place 2 inches apart on parchment paper lined cookie sheets.
- Bake for 8-10 minutes or until center is just set. Chewy and gooey!

143. Easy Halloween Cookies Recipe

Serving: 15 | Prep: | Cook: 10mins | Ready in:

Ingredients

- 1 (12-ounce) bag white chocolate chips
- 1 tablespoon vegetable shortening
- Ritz crackers
- Creamy or crunchy peanut butter
- Orange candy sprinkles

Direction

- In small, heavy saucepan melt chocolate and shortening together over low heat, stirring until smooth.
- Make sandwich cookies out of the Ritz crackers using peanut butter for the filling.
- Dip each cookie into the melted chocolate mixture and place on waxed paper. Sprinkle with the orange candy sprinkles. Allow to dry at room temperature.
- Store in an air tight container at room temperature.

144. Easy Heart Shaped Cookie Recipe

Serving: 12 | Prep: | Cook: 20mins | Ready in:

Ingredients

- 1 pkg. (16.5 oz.) NESTLÉ® TOLL HOUSE® Refrigerated chocolate chip Cookie Bar Dough
- 1/2 cup NESTLÉ® TOLL HOUSE® Semi-sweet chocolate Morsels

Direction

- Preheat oven to 350° F. Grease 9-inch heart-shaped pan.
- Place whole bar of dough in prepared pan.
- Allow to soften for 5 to 10 minutes.
- Using fingertips, pat dough gently to cover bottom.
- Bake for 17 to 19 minutes or until golden brown.
- Cool in pan on wire rack for 10 minutes; remove to wire rack to cool completely.
- Microwave morsels in small, microwave-safe bowl on HIGH (100%) power for 45 seconds; stir. Microwave at additional 10-second intervals, stirring until smooth. Spread over cookie to within 1-inch of edge.

145. Easy Melt In Your Mouth Shortbread Recipe

Serving: 0 | Prep: | Cook: 2hours | Ready in:

Ingredients

- 1 cup softened butter
- 1/2 cup icing sugar
- i/4 cup cornstarch
- 1 1/2 cup flour

Direction

- Cream butter till light and fluffy
- Mix in other ingredient
- Roll into small balls 2cm in diameter and place on an ungreased cookie sheet, bake at 300 degrees F for 10-15 min till slightly browned.
- Awesome drizzled with chocolate

146. Easy Peanut Butter Cake Cookies Recipe

Serving: 36 | Prep: | Cook: 12mins |Ready in:

Ingredients

- 1 pkg yellow cake mix
- 1 cup crunchy peanutbutter
- 1/2 cup canola
- 2 Tbs water
- 2 eggs

Direction

- Mix peanut butter, oil, water and eggs together
- Stir in cake mix well
- Drop by heaping Tbsp. onto cookie sheet
- Using a fork dipped in water, flatter cookies and make a crisscross pattern on them
- Bake 350F about 12 mins.
- Let cool 2 mins on pan before carefully removing

147. Easy Peanut Butter Cookies Recipe

Serving: 1 | Prep: | Cook: 10mins |Ready in:

Ingredients

- 1 cup peanut butter (I use crunchy but smooth is ok too)
- 1 egg
- 1 cup sugar

Direction

- Mix all in a mixing bowl. Spoon them out onto a cookie sheet, making balls. Take a fork and lightly press onto the cookie, making lines from the fork. Turn the cookie sheet 90 degrees and do the same thing again with the fork. The

results should be somewhat of a tic-tac-toe board on top of the cookies.
- Place in the oven and bake for 10 mins at 375 deg. Fahrenheit.
- Take them out when they are turning golden brown, depending on how well done you like your cookies.

148. Easy Peanut Butter Cookies Recipe

Serving: 10 | Prep: | Cook: 9mins |Ready in:

Ingredients

- 1 egg
- 1 cup sugar
- 1 cup peanut butter

Direction

- Combine all ingredients until mixed.
- Roll mixture into 1 inch balls.
- Place on ungreased cookie sheet and flatten each ball with a fork.
- Bake at 350F for 8-10 minutes.
- Cool for 5-7 minutes then place on wire rack.

149. Easy Peppermint Meringues Recipe

Serving: 36 | Prep: | Cook: 90mins |Ready in:

Ingredients

- 8 egg whites
- 1/8 teaspoon salt
- 1/8 teaspoon cream of tartar
- 1/2 cup sugar
- 2 peppermint candy canes, crushed

Direction

- In a mixing bowl, beat egg whites until foamy.
- Sprinkle with salt and cream of tartar; beat until soft peaks form.
- Gradually add sugar, beating until stiff peaks form, about 7 minutes.
- Drop by teaspoonful onto ungreased foil or paper-lined baking sheets; sprinkle with the crushed candy.
- Bake at 225° for 1-1/2 hours.
- Turn off heat; leave cookies in the oven with the door ajar for at least 1 hour or until cool. Store in an airtight container.
- Yield: 3 dozen.

---

150. Eatmore Bars Recipe

Serving: 24 | Prep: | Cook: | Ready in:

Ingredients

- 1 cup peanut butter
- 1 cup corn syrup
- 1 cup chocolate chips
- 3 cups Rice Krispies
- 1 cup peanuts, chopped

Direction

- Grease 8x8 inch pan
- 1.) Put peanut butter, corn syrup and chocolate chips into a medium to large sized pot.
- 2.) Cook over medium heat until everything is melted together. You don't need to boil these.
- 3.) Remove from heat and add peanuts & Krispies.
- 4.) Pour into 8x8 inch pan. Let cool, and voila!

---

151. Egg Yolk Butter Cookies Recipe

Serving: 15 | Prep: | Cook: 1hours10mins | Ready in:

Ingredients

- 300g all-purpose flour
- 6 egg yolks
- 2/3 cup white sugar
- 10g vanilla sugar
- 226g butter

Direction

- Put all ingredients in a food processor and make a dough. Put in a drop of water if the dough don't come together well.
- Form a log of ~8cm diameter, cover with food wrap and put it in a freezer for 30-40 minutes.
- Cut into 0.6cm thick pieces. [0.2in]
- Bake in a preheated [180C - 356F] oven for 12-15 minutes.

---

152. Eggnog Shortbread Recipe

Serving: 4 | Prep: | Cook: 60mins | Ready in:

Ingredients

- 2 sticks unsalted butter, softened
- 3/4 cup powdered sugar, sifted
- 1 T sherry
- 2 cups flour
- 1 t salt
- 1 T freshly grated nutmeg
- About 1/4 cup eggnog
- About 1/4 cup turbinado sugar, for sprinkling (a type of raw sugar with coarse crystals

Direction

- Beat butter and powdered sugar with an electric mixer on high speed until fluffy.
- Add sherry, flour, salt and nutmeg.
- Beat with an electric mixer.
- Mixture will be crumbly and appear dry.
- Continue to mix until a cohesive dough forms, or stop mixer and gently knead into a dough.

- Roll out between 2 sheets of parchment to a thickness of 1/4 inch (about a 10-inch circle).
- Refrigerate for 30 minutes.
- Preheat oven to 325 degrees.
- Cut dough into rounds or other shapes.
- Place 1/2 inch apart on an ungreased cookie sheet.
- Brush with eggnog, sprinkle with sugar and bake for about 15 to 20 minutes.
- Reroll dough scraps and repeat with refrigerating, cutting and baking.
- Store in an airtight container for up to a week.

153. Emerils Awesome Caramel Ice Cream Oatmeal Raisin Cookie Sandwich Recipe

Serving: 1 | Prep: | Cook: |Ready in:

Ingredients

- caramel ice cream oatmeal-Raisin cookie Sandwich
- Recipe courtesy Emeril Lagasse, 2007.
- 2 scoops caramel ice cream, divided
- 2 oatmeal-raisin cookies
- Melted white chocolate, for garnish
- Raspberry sauce, for garnish
- fresh raspberries, for garnish
- Place 1 scoop ice cream between the 2 cookies.
- Paint a serving plate with the melted white chocolate and drizzle with the raspberry sauce.
- Place the other scoop of ice cream on the painted plate.
- Place the ice cream sandwich on top of the ice cream and garnish with the raspberries.
- Yield: 1 ice cream sandwich (Make as many as you like:)

Direction

- PLEASE SEE ALL ABOVE.
- EASY and DELICIOUS!!

154. Excelent Chocolate Chip Cookies Recipe

Serving: 24 | Prep: | Cook: 11mins |Ready in:

Ingredients

- 1 1/2 c. sifted all purpose flour
- 1 t. baking soda
- 1 t. ground cinnamon
- 2 sticks butter (soft)
- 1/2 c. firmly packed brown sugar
- 1 c. sugar
- 1 egg
- 2 1/2 t. vinilla
- 1 c. semi chocolate chips

Direction

- Mix flour, soda, cinnamon
- Beat butter, brown sugar, sugar until fluffy. Then beat in egg and vanilla
- Beat in flour mixture. Fold in chocolate chips and cover and chill for 1hr.
- Preheat oven to 350 F. and grease 2 cookie sheets
- Shape dough into 1 in. balls 2 in, apart and flatten

155. Exquisite Peanut Butter Bars Recipe

Serving: 16 | Prep: | Cook: 10mins |Ready in:

Ingredients

- 1 cup butter
- 1-3/4 cup graham cracker crumbs
- 2-1/2 cups powdered sugar
- 1 cup smooth peanut butter
- 12 ounces chocolate chips

Direction

- Mix all ingredients except chips and press into rectangular baking dish.
- Melt chocolate chips and spread on top of peanut butter mixture.
- Refrigerate to set chocolate then cut into bars and serve.

---

156.   Flourless Almond Butter Cookies Recipe

Serving: 12 | Prep: | Cook: 15mins | Ready in:

Ingredients

- 1 cup of almond butter, room temperature
- 1/2 cup brown sugar
- 1 tsp baking soda
- 1 tsp vanilla
- 1 egg
- Spreadable seedless fruit, I used raspberry
- optional powdered sugar

Direction

- Combine everything except the spreadable fruit.
- Blend well with electric beater till a dough forms.
- Form dough into walnut size balls, you should get at least 12 balls
- Use your finger to form a centre indentation in dough to hold the filling
- Place cookies on a greased cookie sheet a few inches apart
- Fill centre with some of the fruit (about 1/2 tsp. fruit for each cookie)
- Bake in a preheated 325F oven about 15 minutes or set and browned
- Let cool on cookie sheet a few minutes before carefully removing to a wire rack to cool.
- Cookies will harden as they cool.
- Dust with powdered sugar if desired

---

157.   Flourless Peanut Butter Chocolate Chip Cookies Recipe

Serving: 12 | Prep: | Cook: 12mins | Ready in:

Ingredients

- 1 c. chunky peanut butter
- 1 c. packed golden brown sugar (although 1/2 c. is sweet enough for us!)
- 1 lg. egg (or egg substitute)
- 1 t. baking soda
- 1/2 t. pure vanilla extract
- 6 oz. chopped semi-sweet chocolate (or chips)

Direction

- Preheat oven to 350 & mix first 5 ingredients in medium bowl
- Mix in chocolate chunks
- Using moistened fingers form 1 T. cookie balls
- Arrange on 2 ungreased baking sheets 2" apart
- Bake cookies until puffed & golden on bottom about 12 minutes
- Cool on sheets for 5 minutes & transfer to racks until completely cool.
- These are wonderful ~ enjoy!

---

158.   Fortune Cookies Recipe

Serving: 36 | Prep: | Cook: 60mins | Ready in:

Ingredients

- 36 - 1/2 x 2 1/2 inch strips of paper for fortunes
- 3 egg whites
- 1/4 c. granulated sugar
- 1/8 tsp. salt
- 1/2 c. butter or margarine
- 1/2 c. all-purpose flour
- 2 tsp. almond extract
- ------------------------------

- Fortunes:
- - Prosperity is just around the corner.
- - You will meet a tall, dark, handsome, stranger.
- - Do not pretend to be what you do not intend to be.
- - He who laughs hardest, laughs last.
- - Imagination is greater than knowledge.
- - You will travel far in life.
- - He who hesitates is lost.
- - Progress is in the reach of of all who wish to make it.
- - Happiness is sitting right next to you.
- - You will soon discover a new talent.

Direction

- Write fortunes on strips of paper and fold in half; set aside. You can also use your computer and trim them down to size.
- Preheat the oven to 350 degrees F. Beat egg whites until frothy. Beat in sugar and salt. Stir in butter, flour, and almond extract.
- Making no more than six cookies at a time, drop batter by rounded teaspoonful onto ungreased baking sheet about 3 inches apart. Bake 8 to 10 minutes or until edges are light golden brown.
- Working quickly, while cookies are still warm and pliable, hold each cookie in palm and place a fortune on one half of cookie. Fold cookie in half over fortune. Drape the center of the folded cookie over the handle of a wooden spoon. Fold the edges of the cookie around spoon until sides touch; slide off spoon. Repeat with remaining cookies.
- If cookies become brittle before they're shaped, return the pan to the oven for 1 minute to soften. Store in airtight container.

159.   Frosted Lemon Cookies Recipe

Serving: 0 | Prep: | Cook: 45mins | Ready in:

Ingredients

- 2 1/2 cups flour
- 1 1/2 cups sugars
- 1 cup butter, softened
- 2 eggs
- 1 tbsp lemon peel
- 1 tbsp lemon juice
- 1 1/2 tsp cream of tartar
- 1 tsp baking soda
- 1/4 tsp salt
- Glaze: 2 1/2 cups powdered sugar
- 1/4 cup lemon juice
- grated lemon peel

Direction

- Heat the oven to 400 F
- Combine all the cookie ingredients in a large bowl.
- Beat at low speed, scraping the bowl often, until well mixed.
- Drop the dough by rounded teaspoonfuls 2 inches apart onto ungreased cookie sheets.
- Bake at 6 to 8 minutes or until the edges are lightly browned.
- Meanwhile, combine all the glaze ingredients in a small bowl.
- Stir until smooth.
- Frost the warm cookies with the glaze.
- Sprinkle with the grated lemon peel, if desired

160.   Fruit Coctail Bars Recipe

Serving: 2212 | Prep: | Cook: 22mins | Ready in:

Ingredients

- 1 1/2 cups sugar
- 2 eggs
- 1 can (17oz) fruit cocktail, undrained
- 1 tsp. vanilla extract
- 2 1/4 cups all-purpose flour
- 1 /2 tsp. baking soda
- 1 tsp. salt

- 1 1/3 cups flaked coconut
- 1 cup chopped walnuts
- glaze
- 1/2 cup sugar
- 1/4 cup butter or margarine
- 2 tbs. milk
- 1/4 tsp. vanilla extract

Direction

- In a mixing bowl, cream sugar and eggs.
- Add fruit cocktail and vanilla, mix well.
- Combine the flour, baking soda and salt; add to the creamed mixture and mix well.
- Pour into a greased 15-in x 10-in x 1-in baking pan
- Sprinkle with coconut and walnuts.
- Bake at 350 for 20 to 25 minutes or until cake tests done.
- Cool for 10 minutes
- In a saucepan, bring sugar, butter and milk to a boil.
- Remove from the heat'; add vanilla and mix well.
- Drizzle over cake
- Cool, cut into bars.

161. Fruit Pizza Recipe

Serving: 12 | Prep: | Cook: 20mins | Ready in:

Ingredients

- 1 (18 ounce) package refrigerated sugar cookie dough
- 1 (7 ounce) jar marshmallow creme
- 1 (8 ounce) package cream cheese, softened
- fruit of your choice (Examples: kiwi, bananas, strawberries, grapes, mango, etc)

Direction

- Preheat oven to 350 degrees F.
- On an ungreased medium baking sheet, smooth the refrigerated sugar cookie dough

into a single layer approximately 1/4 inch thick. (Dough will be a little stiff – I recommend using a rolling pin and a little bit of flour to help with this.) Bake in the preheated oven 10 minutes, or until edges are lightly browned and center is no longer doughy.

- In a medium bowl, blend the marshmallow crème and cream cheese. Spread the mixture over the baked crust. Decorate "pizza" with your choice of cut-up fruit toppings. Cover and chill in the refrigerator until serving.

162. Fruity Cookies Recipe

Serving: 20 | Prep: | Cook: 10mins | Ready in:

Ingredients

- 3 Very Ripe bananas (Mashed)
- 1/3 Cup applesauce
- 2 Cups rolled oats
- 1/3 Cup wheat germ
- 2 TBS cinnamon
- 1 TBS vanilla extract
- 1 TBS almond extract (optional)
- 2 TBS honey
- 1 Cup Dried and fresh fruits (whatever combo you have handy)

Direction

- Preheat oven to 325F
- In large bowl mash bananas.
- Combine everything else mix well and let stand for 15 min
- Drop onto cookie sheet (do not grease)
- Flatten with back of spoon (they don't spread)
- Bake 10 min
- Cool and enjoy!

163. Fudge Cookies Recipe

Serving: 16 | Prep: | Cook: 15mins | Ready in:

Ingredients

- 3/4 cups of semi-sweet chocolate chips
- 1/2 stick of butter at room temperature
- 1 egg
- 1 tsp. vanilla extract
- 1/3 cup of white sugar
- 1/2 cup of almond flour
- 1/2 tsp. baking powder
- 2 TB unsweetened cocoa powder
- a pinch salt
- 1/3 cup walnuts, chopped or pieces
- 1/2 cup semi-sweet chocolate chips
- 1/2 cup raisins (I use golden raisins.)
- You can buy almond flour which is just powdered almonds at any high quality market or health food store. It adds a chewiness to any cookie, brownie or cake recipe. (I use Bob's Red Mill almond flour.) *You can also substitute 1/2 cup of regular flour if you don't want a gluten-free cookie.
- *You can substitute dried cranberries for the raisins and change the walnuts to pecans.

Direction

- Melt butter and 1/2 c. chips in microwave for 1 1/2 minute.
- Stir well until smooth.
- In medium bowl whisk egg, extract, and sugar until well-combined.
- Stir in the melted chocolate mixture.
- In a separate bowl combine the almond flour, baking powder and salt.
- Mix in with chocolate mixture until barely mixed. .
- Mix in the remaining 1/2 c. chips, nuts, and raisins.
- Cover and chill for one hour.
- Place by tablespoonfuls on greased cookie sheets, then press down each cookie lightly with the back of a spoon.
- Bake at 325 degrees for 13-15 minutes.

- Remove from oven when slightly puffy.
- The cookies will firm up while they cool.

164. Fusion Cookies Recipe

Serving: 20 | Prep: | Cook: 12mins | Ready in:

Ingredients

- ¼ cup shortening
- ¾ cup tahini (sesame butter)
- ½ cup packed brown sugar
- 1 egg
- 1 tsp vanilla
- 2/3 cup flour
- ½ cup whole-wheat flour
- ½ teaspoon baking powder
- ¾ teaspoon baking soda
- 4 tbsp toasted sesame seeds
- ¼ cup diced, dried apple
- 2 tbsp dried cherries

Direction

- Preheat oven to 350F. Lightly grease two baking sheets.
- Cream shortening, tahini, and sugar.
- Add egg and vanilla, beat well.
- Stir together flours, baking powder, baking soda, and sesame seeds.
- Fold in the apple and cherries to the creamed mixture until well blended.
- Drop by spoonfuls on prepared baking sheets.
- Bake 11 minutes. Cool 2 minutes on sheets, then remove to wire rack and cool completely.

165. Germaoodles Recipe

Serving: 24 | Prep: | Cook: 12mins | Ready in:

Ingredients

- 1 box German chocolate cake mix

- 1/2 cup applesauce
- 2 eggs
- 1/2 cup coconut

Direction

- Mix all ingredients.
- Drop onto lightly greased cookie sheets.
- Bake at 350 degrees for 12-14 minutes.

---

166.   Ginger Pumpkin Praline Squares Recipe

Serving: 15 | Prep: | Cook: 40mins | Ready in:

Ingredients

- Filling Ingredients:
- 1 cup firmly packed brown sugar
- 1/4 cup sugar
- 1 (29-ounce) can pumpkin
- 1 (12-ounce) can evaporated milk
- 5 eggs
- 2 teaspoons ground cinnamon
- 1/2 teaspoon ground ginger
- 1/2 teaspoon ground cloves
- Topping Ingredients:
- 3/4 cup all-purpose flour
- 1/2 cup firmly packed brown sugar
- 1/4 cup cold LAND O LAKES® butter
- 1/2 cup chopped pecans

Direction

- Garnish Ingredients:
- LAND O LAKES™ Heavy Whipping Cream, whipped, sweetened, if desired
- Ground cinnamon, if desired
- Preparation:
- Heat oven to 350°F. Combine all filling ingredients in large bowl. Beat at medium speed, scraping bowl often, until smooth.
- Pour into greased 13x9-inch baking pan. Bake for 25 to 30 minutes or until partially set.

- Meanwhile, combine 3/4 cup flour and 1/2 cup brown sugar in small bowl; cut in butter with pastry blender or fork until mixture resembles coarse crumbs. Stir in pecans. Sprinkle topping over hot, partially baked pumpkin filling. Continue baking for 15 to 20 minutes or until knife inserted in centre comes out clean. Cool 30 minutes. Refrigerate until cooled completely (1 1/2 hours).
- To serve, dollop each serving with whipped cream; sprinkle with cinnamon, if desired. Store refrigerated.

---

167.   Gingerbread People Recipe

Serving: 212 | Prep: | Cook: 15mins | Ready in:

Ingredients

- 1 1/2 cups dark molasses
- 1 cup packed brown sugar
- 2/3 cup cold water
- 1/3 cup shortening
- 7 cups all purpose flour
- 2 teaspoons baking soda
- 1 teaspoon salt
- 1 teaspoon ground allspice
- 1 teaspoon ground ginger
- 2 teaspoons ground cloves
- 1 teaspoon cinnamon

Direction

- Mix molasses brown sugar, water and shortening
- Mix in remaining ingredients
- Cover and refrigerate at least 2 hours
- Heat oven to 350F
- Roll dough 1/4 inch thick on floured board
- Cut with floured gingerbread cutter or favorite cutter
- Place about 2 inches apart on lightly greased cookie sheet
- 10-12 min cool

- Put frosting to decorate

168. Glazed Doughnut Crips Cookies Recipe

Serving: 16 | Prep: | Cook: 12mins | Ready in:

Ingredients

- COOKIE:
- 1 (18-once) package refrigerated sugar cookie dough, room temperature
- (recommended: Pilsbury)
- 1/2 cup all purpose flour
- 1/2 teaspoon brandy extract (or flavored extract of your choice)
- Prepared vanilla frosting
- drippy icing, recipe follows
- DRIPPY ICING:
- 1 cup sifted powdered sugar
- 2 tablespoons milk
- 1 drop yellow food coloring

Direction

- COOKIES:
- Knead dough with flour, adding in 2 parts, and brandy extract. Break into 2-inch pieces. Roll each piece into a 6-inch long rope. On an ungreased cookie sheet, shape rope like a doughnut, pinching ends together. Freeze for 10 minutes. Bake for 10 - 12 minutes. Cookies should be just lightly golden on top.
- Cool completely. Frost each cookie with vanilla frosting. Drizzle Drippy Icing over cookies.
- DRIPPY ICING:
- In a small bowl, whisk together powdered sugar and milk. Tint with 1 drop yellow food coloring. Add more powdered sugar for a stiffer consistency, if desired.
- Drizzle over cookies.

169. Golden Raisin Cookies Recipe

Serving: 0 | Prep: | Cook: 20mins | Ready in:

Ingredients

- 1 cup butter, softened
- 1 1/2 cups sugar
- 1 tbsp lemon juice
- 2 eggs
- 3 1/2 cups flour
- 1 1/2 tsp cream of tartar
- 1 1/2 tsp baking soda
- 1 pkg (15 oz.) golden raisins (2 1/2 cups)

Direction

- In a large bowl, cream the butter and the sugar until light and fluffy.
- Add the lemon juice and the eggs
- Combine the dry ingredients
- Gradually add to the creamed mixture
- Stir in the raisins
- Roll into 1-inch balls
- Place on greased baking sheets
- Flatten with a floured fork
- Bake at 400 for 8 to 10 minutes or until lightly browned

170. Graham Cracker Bars Recipe

Serving: 15 | Prep: | Cook: 5mins | Ready in:

Ingredients

- 30 whole graham crackers
- 2 sticks butter
- 1 cup granulated sugar
- 1/2 cup milk
- 1 egg well beaten
- 1/2 cup coconut
- 1 cup chopped pecans
- 1 cup graham cracker crumbs

- Frosting:
- 1 stuck butter softened
- 6 tablespoons evaporated milk
- 2 cups powdered sugar sifted
- 1 teaspoon vanilla
- 1/2 cup finely chopped pecans
- 1 cup coconut

Direction

- Line bottom of a rectangular baking pan with a layer of whole graham crackers. Combine melted butter, sugar, milk and beaten egg in a saucepan then cook over medium heat stirring constantly until mixture comes to a boil. Remove from heat and add coconut, nuts and crumbs. Spread over crackers. Top with remaining crackers. To make frosting combine butter, milk, sugar, vanilla and pecans and beat until smooth. Spread on top of graham crackers and refrigerate for 24 hours. Sprinkle with coconut then cut into bars and serve.

171.   Grandma's Mmmmmm Peanutbutter Cookies Recipe

Serving: 0 | Prep: | Cook: 14mins | Ready in:

Ingredients

- 1 cup butter flavored shortening
- 1 cup sugar
- 1 cup firmly packed brown sugar
- 1 teaspoon vanilla extract
- 2 eggs
- 1 1/2 cups peanut butter
- 2 cups all-purpose flour
- 2 teaspoons baking soda
- 1 teaspoon salt

Direction

- 1 Preheat oven to 350
- 2 Cream shortening, sugars, and vanilla extract.

- 3 Add eggs, and beat thoroughly.
- 4 Stir in peanut butter.
- 5 Combine dry ingredients; stir into creamed mixture.
- 6 Using ice cream scoop, place 6 level scoops on ungreased cookie sheet
- 7 Press with back of fork dipped in sugar to make a crisscross design.
- 8 Bake at 350° 14 minutes.
- 9 Remove from oven & let cool on cookie sheet for at least 5 minutes. Then transfer to wire cooling rack until completely cool.

172.   Grandma's Pecan Balls Recipe

Serving: 0 | Prep: | Cook: 1hours | Ready in:

Ingredients

- 1 cup butter, softened
- 5 tbsp sugar
- 2 tsp vanilla
- 2 cups flour
- 2 cups pecans, broken
- Gransih: powdered sugar

Direction

- In a medium bowl, blend together the butter and sugar.
- Stir in the vanilla and the flour.
- Fold in the pecans.
- Roll the dough into walnut-size balls
- Arrange on an ungreased baking sheet.
- Bake at 300oF for 45 minutes.
- While warm, sprinkle the cookies with powdered sugar
- Sprinkle again before serving.

173. Grandpas Figgy Cookies Recipe

Serving: 40 | Prep: | Cook: 20mins | Ready in:

Ingredients

- Filling
- 2/3 cup diced dried figs
- 1/3 cup grape or orange juice
- 1/3 cup unsweetened applesauce
- 4 tsp lemon juice
- 2 tsp ground cinnamon
- Dough
- 1/3 cup all purpose flour
- 3/4 cup whole wheat flour
- 1/4 cup brown sugar
- 1/2 tsp baking powder
- 1/4 tsp baking soda
- 1/4 tsp ground cinnamon
- 1/4 tsp salt
- 1/3 cup shortening
- 1 egg
- 1 egg yolk
- 1 egg white mixed with 2 Tbsp water for egg wash

Direction

- Combine all filling ingredients in a small saucepot and bring up to a simmer.
- Simmer until the figs absorb all liquid, about 15 minutes.
- Let cool and purée in a food processor before chilling completely.
- Combine flour, sugar, baking powder, baking soda, cinnamon and salt.
- Cut in shortening until dough is a coarse mealy texture.
- Add whole egg and egg yolk and blend in until dough comes together.
- Shape into a disc, wrap and chill for an hour.
- Preheat oven to 375 °F.
- On a lightly floured surface, roll out dough into a rectangle, just under ¼-inch thick.
- Using a knife or pastry cutter, cut strips of dough that are about 5 inches wide.
- Spoon filling along center of each strip. Don't over-fill!
- Brush one side of pastry dough with egg wash and fold the other side of pastry over filling, so that egg washed side meets it.
- Trim edges.
- Lift filled cookie tube to a greased or lined baking sheet and press down to flatten slightly.
- Repeat with remaining strips.
- Brush tops with egg wash.
- Bake for 15 to 18 minutes, until a light golden brown.
- Cool cookies on sheets before cutting the bars strips into bites.

174. Grape Nuts Pb Bars Recipe

Serving: 30 | Prep: | Cook: 10mins | Ready in:

Ingredients

- 3/4 cup peanut butter
- 1 cup light corn syrup
- 1 cup sugar
- 4 cups Grape-Nuts cereal

Direction

- Spray 9x13 pan with a non-stick spray and set aside.
- .Microwave peanut butter, corn syrup and sugar in a large microwaveable bowl on high for 2 minutes or until mixture comes to a boil, stirring after each minute.
- Add cereal and mix well.
- Press mixture into firmly onto bottom of 9x13 pan and cool completely.
- Cut into bars and serve.

175. Great Great Grammas Empire Cookies Recipe

Serving: 16 | Prep: | Cook: 10mins | Ready in:

Ingredients

- 1 c butter
- 1/2 c brown sugar
- 1/2 c white sugar
- 1 tsp baking soda
- 2 tsp cream of tartar
- 1 egg
- 3 c all-purpose flour

Direction

- Cream together butter and sugars.
- Add egg and blend.
- Combine flour, cream of tartar, and baking soda then stir into sugar mixture.
- For into a shaggy dough ball and turn out onto counter and knead for about 5 minutes or until dough comes together.
- Roll and cut desired shapes then bake in a 350 oven for 10 minutes or until golden brown.
- Cool on racks.
- Great Gramma's instructions when she wrote out this recipe said simply: "Mix it all together and knead it if you have time." :)

176. Green Pumpkinseed And Cranberry Crispy Bars Recipe

Serving: 16 | Prep: | Cook: 10mins | Ready in:

Ingredients

- cooking spray
- 1/2 cup raw green pumpkinseeds
- 1/4 cup butter $
- 1 (8-ounce) package miniature marshmallows (about 5 cups)
- 1 teaspoon vanilla extract
- 1/8 teaspoon salt $
- 5 cups oven-toasted rice cereal (such as rice Krispies) $
- 1 cup dried cranberries

Direction

- Heat a large non-stick skillet over medium-high heat. Coat pan with cooking spray. Add pumpkinseeds; cook 4 minutes or until seeds begin to pop and lightly brown, stirring frequently. Remove from heat; cool.
- Lightly coat a 13 x 9-inch baking dish with cooking spray; set aside. Melt butter in a large saucepan over medium heat. Stir in marshmallows; cook 2 minutes or until smooth, stirring constantly. Remove from heat; stir in vanilla and salt. Stir in reserved seeds, cereal, and cranberries. Scrape mixture into prepared dish using a rubber spatula.
- Lightly coat hands with cooking spray; press cereal mixture evenly into prepared dish. Cool completely. Cut into 16 bars.
- Nutritional Information
- Amount per serving
- Calories: 152
- Calories from fat: 29%
- Fat: 4.9g
- Saturated fat: 2.2g
- Monounsaturated fat: 1.4g
- Polyunsaturated fat: 1g
- Protein: 1.9g
- Carbohydrate: 26.3g
- Fiber: 0.7g
- Cholesterol: 7.5mg
- Iron: 0.9mg
- Sodium: 115mg
- Calcium: 4.7mg

177. Heavenly Pineapple Fluff Squares Recipe

Serving: 12 | Prep: | Cook: 180mins | Ready in:

Ingredients

- 2 1/4 cups graham cracker crumbs
- 1/2 cup melted butter, do not use margarine
- 1/2 cup softened butter, do not use margarine
- 1 1/2 cups icing sugar
- 2 unbeaten eggs
- 1 pint whipping cream
- 2 cups crushed pineapple, well drained

Direction

- Mix the graham wafer crumbs with the melted butter and spread the mixture in a greased 9 X 13 glass baking pan. Reserve a small amount to sprinkle on top.
- Bake for 15 minutes at 350°, remove from oven and cool completely.
- Mix the softened butter, icing sugar, and eggs, and beat well, till smooth and creamy.
- Spread mixture over the cooled crumb crust.
- Whip the cream till slightly stiff peaks form, then gently blend the drained pineapple into the whipped cream.
- Spread on top of the icing sugar mixture, and sprinkle with remaining crumbs and chill at least 3 hours before serving.

178.   Hippie Cookies Recipe

Serving: 48 | Prep: | Cook: 10mins | Ready in:

Ingredients

- 1 cup butter
- 3/4 cup brown sugar
- 3/4 cups white sugar
- 1 tsp vanilla
- 2 eggs
- 1 c whole wheat flour
- 1 c white flour
- 1 tsp each baking powder and soda
- 1 cup coconut
- 1 cup oatmeal
- 1 cup Rice Krispies
- 1 cup raisins (or any small bite dried fruit)
- 1 cup chocolate chips

- 3/4 cup sunflower seeds
- 1/3 cup wheat germ
- 1/3 cup chopped nuts
- oven 350 degrees

Direction

- In large bowl mix / beat butter, sugars, vanilla and eggs
- Add flours, baking powder and baking soda in another bowl and blend well.
- Add the flour mixture to the butter mixture. Give a little stir
- Add all remaining ingredients making sure it is nice and bended
- Roll into balls, flatten with a fork and bake 10 minutes.
- Depending on size can make up to 5 dozen

179.   Homemade Twix Bars Recipe

Serving: 15 | Prep: | Cook: 5mins | Ready in:

Ingredients

- Club crackers
- 1 cup of club cracker crumbs
- 1 stick butter
- 3/4 cup brown sugar
- 1/2 cup of granulated sugar
- 1/3 cup milk
- 1 cup chocolate chips
- 3/4 cup peanut butter

Direction

- Line a 9x13 inch pan with whole crackers.
- Boil butter, cracker crumbs, sugars, and milk.
- Cook for 5 minutes.
- Pour over crackers.
- Add another layer of crackers.
- Melt chocolate and peanut butter together.
- Spread over crackers.
- Allow to cool, and then serve.

180. Honey Almond Bars Recipe

Serving: 9 | Prep: | Cook: 40mins | Ready in:

Ingredients

- 3/4 cup of unsalted butter
- 1 cup of all purpose flour
- 1/3 cup of honey
- 1 cup of sliced almonds
- 1/2 cup of sifted confectioner's sugar
- 1/4 tsp of salt
- 2 tsp of lemon juice
- 1/2 tsp of almond extract

Direction

- In a large bowl, cream together 1/2 cup of the butter and the confectioner's sugar.
- Stir in flour and salt.
- Pat evenly into an ungreased 9 inch square cake pan.
- Bake in 350 degree oven for 12 to 15 minutes or until lightly golden.
- Meanwhile, in a small saucepan, melt remaining butter.
- Stir in honey and lemon juice.
- Bring to a boil over medium high heat, stirring constantly.
- Remove from heat.
- Stir in almonds and almond extract.
- Spread evenly over hot baked layer and return to oven for about 15 minutes until evenly golden brown.
- While hot, cut in squares, allow to cool in pan.

181. Honey Lemon Cookies Recipe

Serving: 12 | Prep: | Cook: 15mins | Ready in:

Ingredients

- 1/3 cup butter softened
- 1/2 cup granulated sugar
- 1/2 cup honey
- 1 egg
- 1 teaspoon grated lemon zest
- 2-1/4 cups flour
- 1/2 cup wheat germ divided
- 1 teaspoon baking powder
- 1/4 teaspoon salt

Direction

- In a mixing bowl cream butter and sugar.
- Beat in honey, egg and lemon zest.
- Combine flour, 1/4 cup wheat germ, baking powder and salt then gradually add to creamed mixture.
- Cover and refrigerate for 1 hour.
- Roll dough into balls and roll in remaining wheat germ.
- Place 2 inches apart on baking sheets coated with non-stick cooking spray.
- Bake at 350 for 12 minutes then remove to wire racks to cool.

182. Irresistable Choc Chunk Cookies Recipe

Serving: 12 | Prep: | Cook: 30mins | Ready in:

Ingredients

- 1 cup butter
- 3/4 cup sugar
- 2/3 cup brown sugar
- 1 egg
- 3 tsp vanilla
- 1 1/2 tbsp whole milk or cream
- 1 tsp cinnamon
- 1 2/3 cups flour
- 1 1/4 tsp baking soda
- 1 tsp baking powder
- 1/2 tsp salt

- 1/2 cup ground oats (optional but really nice)
- 1 1/2 cups chocolate chunks

Direction

- Cream butter and sugars
- Add egg, vanilla, milk and mix
- Add dry ingredients except chocolate and mix
- Add chocolate and mix
- Bake at 250 for 8 minutes or until crispy on the outside and soft in the middle.

183.   Italian Cookies Recipe

Serving: 25 | Prep: | Cook: 8mins | Ready in:

Ingredients

- For the cookies:
- 1/2 cup butter
- 1/4 cup shortening
- 3/4 cup granulated sugar
- 4 eggs
- 3 cups all-purpose flour
- 5 teaspoons baking powder
- 1/2 teaspoon table salt
- 2 teaspoons anise extract (okay to use vanilla or lemon)
- For the glaze
- 3-4 Tablespoons milk
- 2 cups powdered sugar
- 1 teaspoon anise extract

Direction

- Sift flour, baking powder and salt together in a bowl. Set aside.
- In the microwave melt butter and shortening (make sure the shortening is fresh or it will taste bad) together in a bowl.
- Beat the melted butter and shortening together until it is completely incorporated, about 2 minutes. Add granulated sugar and mix well. Add eggs, one at a time, beating well after

each addition, about 1 minute each. Mix in anise extract.
- Add the flour mixture to the creamed mixture slowly, until fully incorporated. Don't over mix. If the cookie dough is too sticky to roll in the palm of your hand, add a bit of flour. However, the dough should remain very soft, so don't add too much.
- Roll the cookie dough in small balls (they puff up quite nicely) and place them on ungreased cookie sheets. Bake at 375 degrees for 8-10 minutes (mine took 8 minutes). The bottoms of the cookies should be lightly browned but the tops of should remain light in colour.
- Remove cookies from the cookie sheet immediately and move to a wire rack. Cool completely before glazing.
- For the glaze, slowly mix milk with powdered sugar and anise extract. The glaze needs to be thick to adhere to the cookie. Dip the top of each cookie into the glaze.
- Sprinkle each cookie with nonpareils and leave them to completely dry.
- This recipe made approximately 100 cookies when dough was rolled into 3/4" balls.

184.   Jacques Pépin's Chocolate Chunk Cookies Recipe

Serving: 10 | Prep: | Cook: | Ready in:

Ingredients

- 1 stick unsalted butter, softened
- 2 cage free egg yolks
- 1/2 cup organic sugar
- 1 cup all-purpose flour
- 1/4 teaspoon sea salt
- 2 tablespoons E. Guittard unsweetened cocoa powder
- 1/2 cup Scharffen Berger Semisweet baking chunks

Direction

- Set aside chunks and 1 tablespoon of cinnamon sugar. Mix remaining ingredients with a wooden spoon in bowl (or 30 seconds in food processor) until smooth. Transfer dough to a sheet of plastic wrap and roll into a 10" log, 1" thick. Refrigerate 1 hour.
- Preheat oven to 350°F with rack in center.
- Unwrap cold log and sprinkle evenly with remaining tablespoon of sugar. Cut log into 20 cookies, each 1/2" thick. Press the chunks directly into the cookies. Line a cookie sheet with parchment paper. Arrange cookies 1" apart, chips facing up. Bake 14-15 min. Cool on wire rack.

185. Kasha Kookies Recipe

Serving: 60 | Prep: | Cook: 15mins | Ready in:

Ingredients

- 1 cup toasted buckwheat groats (kasha)
- 1 cup mixed raisins and chopped dates
- 4 cups grape juice
- ¼ teaspoon salt
- ½ cup soybean flour
- ½ cup brown rice flour
- ½ cup whole-wheat pastry flour
- 1 cup rolled oats

Direction

- Preheat oven to 350F. Lightly grease cookie sheets.
- Bring the buckwheat groats, dried fruit and juice to a boil.
- Add salt reduce the heat and cover the pan.
- Simmer for 15 minutes. Uncover and let cool for 15 minutes.
- Combine all the ingredients except the oat flakes in a.
- Form the dough into small balls. (Tip: it helps to dip your fingers in cold water)

- Roll the balls in the oats.
- Place the balls 1 inch apart on the prepared cookie sheet.
- Press down with the moistened tines of a fork.
- Bake for 15 minutes.

186. Key Lime And Macadamia Cornmeal Cookies Recipe

Serving: 0 | Prep: | Cook: 2hours | Ready in:

Ingredients

- 1 stick butter, melted or VERY soft, but cooled
- 1/2 cup honey
- 1 egg
- 1T fresh key lime juice(3-5 key limes, probably)
- zest from all above limes
- 1t rum or vanilla extract
- 1 1/4 cup flour
- 1/2 cup fine cornmeal
- 1/2t salt
- 1/4 cup chopped, roasted, macadamia nuts
- 1/4 cup white chocolate chips or chopped white chocolate
- lime Glaze
- 1 cup confectioners sugar
- 1T key lime juice
- 1-3t water, as needed, to thin to drizzleable consistency

Direction

- Cream butter and honey together until well combined and smooth.
- Add egg and stir well.
- Add lime juice and zest, and rum or vanilla extract and combine well.
- Add flour, cornmeal and salt and mix slowly until well incorporated.
- Fold in nuts and chocolate.

- Spoon dough onto waxed paper and, using the paper, shape dough into a log, about 2 inches in diameter, or, shape into a triangular shape of similar size.
- Refrigerate at least 1 hour and up to overnight.
- Unroll log and slice off cookies, about 1/4-1/2 inch thick, place on ungreased cookie sheet or baking stone, and bake for 12 minutes. Cookies don't really brown, and they don't raise, so 12-13 minutes and the cookies should be set.
- Let cool on baking sheet/stone about 3 minutes then remove to wire rack to cool.
- For Glaze
- Whisk together sugar and lime juice, adding a little water at a time, until a consistency which you can drizzle over cookies. (I use a condiment bottle :)
- Glaze slightly warmed cookies, then let finish cooling.

187.   Kit Kat Bars Recipe

Serving: 1 | Prep: | Cook: |Ready in:

Ingredients

- Ritz crackers
- 1-1/2 c. graham crackers, crushed
- 3/4 c. brown sugar
- 1 c. granulated sugar
- 3/4 c. butter or margarine
- 1/3 c. milk
- 1 tsp. vanilla
- 1 c. butterscotch chips
- 1 c. semisweet chocolate chips
- 3/4 c. smooth peanut butter

Direction

- Put graham crackers, brown sugar, white sugar, butter, milk in a saucepan; bring it to a boil. Boil for 5 minutes. Remove from heat and add vanilla.

- Place a layer of Ritz Crackers in a 13x9" pan and pour 1/2 of the mixture over it. Make another layer of Ritz Crackers and pour the remaining mixture. Add one last row of Ritz Crackers.
- Over low heat, melt both chips and peanut butter. When melted, spread evenly over the top layer of crackers. When cool, cut into desired bars or squares.

188.   Lace Cookies Recipe

Serving: 48 | Prep: | Cook: 7mins |Ready in:

Ingredients

- 1 stick butter
- 1 cup brown sugar
- 1 cup quick oats(uncooked)
- 2 Tablespoons flour
- 1 teaspoon vanilla
- pinch of salt

Direction

- Mix all ingredients and chill
- Roll into little balls about the size of a marble
- Place on cookie sheet FAR apart as they melt down as they cook
- Bake at 375 degrees for about 7 minutes
- Makes about 4 dozen.
- **
- Pray for wisdom, knowledge & understanding
- **

189.   Lemon Almond Biscotti Recipe

Serving: 12 | Prep: | Cook: 60mins |Ready in:

Ingredients

- 2 1/4 cups all purpose flour
- 1/2 cup chopped toasted almonds
- 1 teaspoon baking powder
- 1/2 teaspoon salt
- 1 cup sugar
- 1/2 cup (1 stick) unsalted butter, at room temperature
- 2 large eggs
- 1/4 cup fresh lemon juice
- 1 tablespoon grated lemon peel
- 1 teaspoon vanilla extract
- 1/2 teaspoon almond extract
- 1 large egg white, beaten (for glaze)

Direction

- Preheat oven to 350 degrees.
- Spray heavy large baking sheet with non-stick spray.
- Mix flour and next 3 ingredients in medium bowl.
- Beat sugar and butter in large bowl until light and fluffy. Add eggs 1 at a time, beating well after each addition. Beat in juice, peel and extracts.
- Mix in dry ingredients.
- Turn dough out onto heavily floured surface. Divide in half. Shape each half into an 11 inch long log. Place on baking sheet, spacing 4 inches apart. Flatten each log to width of 1 3/4 inches. Brush with egg white.
- Bake until pale golden, about 30 minutes. Transfer to work surface; cool slightly. Maintain oven temperature.
- Cut each log crosswise on diagonal into 1/2 inches thick slices. Place cookies cut side down on baking sheet.
- Bake until golden, turning once, about 20 minutes.
- Transfer cookies to racks; cool.
- Keep in airtight container for 1 week at room temperature or freeze up to 1 month.

190.   Lemon Bars Recipe

Serving: 20 | Prep: | Cook: 35mins | Ready in:

Ingredients

- 1 C. (2 sticks butter)
- 1 C. sugar
- 2 C. flour
- 1 1/4 C. oatmeal (not instant)
- juice of 3 lemons
- Zest of 2 lemons, chopped fine
- Zest of 1 orange, chopped fine
- 1 (14 oz.) can sweetened condensed milk

Direction

- Cream butter and sugar, then add flour and oatmeal to make dough it will be crumbly). Set aside. Stir juice and zest into milk. Set aside. Butter a 9 x 13 inch pan. Press 2/3 of the dough into the pan. Spread lemon/milk mixture evenly over the top of the dough. Sprinkle the remaining dough over the top. Bake at 350 degrees for 30 to 35 minutes until golden.
- When cool, slice into 1 inch squares.

191.   Lemon Cheesecake Bars Recipe

Serving: 1 | Prep: | Cook: 30mins | Ready in:

Ingredients

- 1 box yellow cake mix (2 layer)
- 8 oz. pkg. cream cheese softened
- 2 eggs
- 1/4 C. sugar
- 1 T. lemon juice
- 1/3 C. vegetable oil

Direction

- Preheat oven to 350. Use a 9x13 baking pan.

- Mix dry cake mix, 1 of the eggs and 1/3 C. oil until crumbly.
- Reserve 1 cup of this mixture for later. Pat the remaining mixture lightly in the pan.
- Bake 15 minutes. While this is baking beat cream cheese, sugar, lemon juice and the remaining egg until light and smooth.
- Spread over baked crumb mixture. Sprinkle reserved crumb mix on top and bake an additional 15 minutes. Be careful not to overbake. Will be light golden brown. Chill thoroughly and cut bars.

192. Lemon Coconut Bites Recipe

Serving: 12 | Prep: | Cook: 1mins | Ready in:

Ingredients

- 1 cup Tropical Traditions coconut cream concentrate
- 3 tablespoons coconut oil
- 1/2 cup honey
- 1 tablespoon lemon zest
- 2 lemons, juiced

Direction

- Place coconut cream concentrate in a medium saucepan over very low heat. Stir constantly until soft and smooth.
- Remove from heat and stir in remaining ingredients until well blended and smooth.
- Place mixture in freezer to firm up (if needed), stirring every few minutes to prevent clumping.
- Line a cookie sheet with parchment paper and with a small cookie scoop, drop mixture unto paper and refrigerate until firm.
- Enjoy!

193. Lemon Cream Cheese Bars Recipe

Serving: 20 | Prep: | Cook: 30mins | Ready in:

Ingredients

- 1 Duncan Hines yellow cake mix with Pudding
- 1 (8oz) pkg. cream cheese
- 1/3 cup sugar
- 1 tsp. lemon juice
- 1/3 cup oil
- 2 eggs

Direction

- Combine dry cake mix with 1/3 cup oil and 1 egg.
- Mix until crumbly.
- Reserve 1 cup and pat remaining mixture lightly in ungreased 13x9x2 inch cake pan.
- Bake at 350 degrees for 15 minutes.
- Beat cream cheese, sugar, lemon and 1 egg until light and smooth.
- Spread over baked layer.
- Sprinkle with the reserved crumbs.
- Bake at 350 degrees for 15 minutes more.
- Cool and cut into bars (16-24).

194. Lemon Cream Cheese Bars Special Recipe

Serving: 10 | Prep: | Cook: 26mins | Ready in:

Ingredients

- Crust:
- 1 box of cake mix (Lemon, butter, Yellow or White)
- 1 1/2 sticks of melted butter (3/4 cup)
- 1/2 cup chopped walnuts (optional)
- Topping:
- 1 8oz. of cream cheese (you can use fat free)

- 2 cups powder sugar (extra for sprinkling after cooked)
- 2 Lg. eggs
- 1 large fresh lemon (1/3 cup juice)
- zest of 1 lemon (optional)

Direction

- Spray 9x13 baking pan, set oven at 350*
- Mix crust ingredients together until crumbly. Press into pan.
- Beat Topping ingredients until smooth. Pour over crust and bake.
- Check after 25 min. when lightly browned and not too jiggly, it will be done.
- Sprinkle with Powdered sugar when cool.

---

195.   Lemon Crisps Recipe

Serving: 48 | Prep: | Cook: 9mins | Ready in:

Ingredients

- 1 box of lemon cake mix
- 1/3 cup oil
- 2 eggs
- sugar
- 1 cup powdered sugar
- juice of 1 lemon

Direction

- Preheat oven to 375 degrees.
- Mix powdered sugar and lemon juice in a bowl until there are no clumps. This will be used when cookies are cooled.
- Mix cake mix, eggs, and oil in bowl with spatula.
- Roll dough into 1-inch balls and place of cookie sheet.
- Pour sugar into a bowl. Dip a flat surface (I use the bottom of a measuring cup) into the sugar and flatten each cookie about 1/4 inch thick. You will probably have to dip the flat surface into the sugar before flattening each cookie.
- Bake for about 9 minutes or until edges are golden brown.
- Let sit on baking sheet for about 2 minutes, then transfer to cooling rack, or just onto wax paper.
- When cookies are cool enough, drizzle powdered sugar and lemon juice mix onto each cookie. You can add sugar crystal sprinkles to add more color if you want.

---

196.   Lemon Dream Bars Recipe

Serving: 1 | Prep: | Cook: 35mins | Ready in:

Ingredients

- 3 C. graham cracker crumbs
- 3/4 C. butter melted
- 1 egg plus 3 egg yolks
- 1 (14 oz) can Eagle Brand sweetened condensed milk(not evaporated)
- 1/2 C. lemon juice

Direction

- Preheat oven to 350.
- In a large bowl mix graham cracker crumbs, butter and lightly beaten egg until combined.
- Reserve one cup of the mixture.
- Press remaining crumb mixture into the bottom of a 9x13" baking dish.
- Bake 10-15 minutes or until lightly toasted.
- With mixer or wire whisk, beat 3 egg yolks, add Eagle Brand and then lemon juice.
- Spread over pressed crumb mixture.
- Top with reserved crumb mixture. Bake 25 minutes longer or until set.
- Cool. Refrigerate 2 hours. Cut into bars.

197. Lemon Hazelnut Logs Recipe

Serving: 36 | Prep: | Cook: 20mins | Ready in:

Ingredients

- 2 cups butter
- 1-1/2 cups light brown sugar
- 2 teaspoons grated lemon rind
- 5 cups flour
- 1/2 teaspoon lemon juice
- 2 egg whites beaten with 2 tablespoons water
- 2 cups hazelnuts finely chopped

Direction

- Preheat oven to 400.
- Cream together butter, brown sugar and lemon rind until fluffy.
- Sift flour and salt together then add to butter mixture.
- Add lemon juice and mix well then chill several hours.
- Shape into fingers about 1-1/2 " long and 1/2" in diameter.
- Roll in egg white beaten with water then roll in chopped nuts and bake 12 minutes.

198. Lemon Hazelnut Squares Recipe

Serving: 16 | Prep: | Cook: 38mins | Ready in:

Ingredients

- Crust:
- 1 cup all-purpose flour
- ¼ cup sugar
- ¼ teaspoon salt
- 6 tablespoons (approx. 3/4 stick) chilled unsalted butter cut into pieces
- ¼ cup shopped husked toasted hazelnuts
- filling:
- ¾ cup sugar

- pinch of salt
- 2 eggs
- 3 tablespoons fresh lemon juice
- 1 tablespoon minced lemon peel (zest)
- ½ teaspoon baking powder

Direction

- For crust: Preheat oven to 350°F.
- Line 8-inch square baking pan with foil; butter foil.
- Mix flour, sugar and salt in food processor.
- Add butter and nuts and blend until fine meal forms.
- Press onto bottom of prepared pan.
- Bake until light brown around edges, about 18 minutes.
- Meanwhile, prepare filling:
- Blend first 6 ingredients in food processor.
- Pour filling onto hot crust.
- Bake until filling begins to brown at edges and is just springy to the touch, about 20 minutes.
- Cool completely in pan on rack.
- Lift foil and dessert from pan.
- Gently peel foil from edges.
- Cut dessert into 16 squares.
- (Can be made one day ahead. Wrap tightly; chill.)
- Sift powdered sugar over lemon squares; serve at room temperature.
- This recipe yields 16 cookies.

199. Lemon Raspberry Cheesecake Bars Recipe

Serving: 30 | Prep: | Cook: 45mins | Ready in:

Ingredients

- Crust:
- Non-stick cooking spray
- 3/4 cup Crisco® butter flavor shortening (or 3/4 stick)
- 1/2 cup firmly packed brown sugar

- 1-1/4 cups all-purpose flour
- 1 cup uncooked oats
- 1/4 teaspoons salt
- Filling:
- 3/4 cup Smucker's® Seedless Red raspberry jam
- 16 ounces cream cheese, softened
- 3/4 cup sugar
- 2 tablespoons all-purpose flour
- 2 large eggs
- 3 tablespoons fresh lemon juice, no seeds please
- 2 teaspoons freshly grated lemon peel

Direction

- Preheat oven to 350°.
- Spray a 13x9x2-inch baking pan with non-stick cooking spray. Set aside.
- Crust:
- In a bowl, combine shortening and brown sugar, beat with an electric mixer at medium speed until well blended.
- Gradually add 1-1/4 cups flour, oats and salt.
- Beat at low speed until well blended.
- Press crust mixture into bottom of prepared pan.
- Bake for 20 minutes or until lightly browned.
- Filling:
- Let crust stand after removing from oven for 2 minutes.
- Spoon raspberry jam onto hot crust.
- Spread carefully to cover.
- In a bowl, combine cream cheese, sugar and 2 tablespoons flour.
- Beat with an electric mixer at low speed until well blended.
- Add eggs and beat again until well blended.
- Add lemon juice and lemon peel. Beat until smooth.
- Pour over the raspberry layer.
- Bake 25 minutes or until set.
- Remove pan and put on wire rack to cool.
- Let cool to room temperature.
- Cut into 30 bars.
- Cover and refrigerate any un-eaten portions.

200.   Lemon Refrigerator Cookies Recipe

Serving: 36 | Prep: | Cook: 10mins | Ready in:

Ingredients

- 3/4 cup granulated sugar
- 3/4 cup packed light brown sugar
- 1 cup unsalted butter softened
- 2 teaspoons lemon extract
- 2 eggs
- 3 cups flour
- 1 tablespoon grated lemon peel
- 1-1/2 teaspoons baking powder
- 3/4 teaspoon salt
- 1 cup finely chopped pecans

Direction

- In large bowl combine sugar, brown sugar, butter, extract and eggs then beat well.
- Add flour, peel, baking powder and salt and blend well then stir in nuts.
- Divide dough into 3 equal parts.
- Shape each into roll and wrap with plastic wrap then refrigerate 2 hours.
- Heat oven to 425 then cut into 1/4" slices.
- Place slices 1" apart on ungreased cookie sheets and bake 7 minutes.
- Remove immediately from cookie sheets and allow to cool on racks.

201.   Lemon Shortbread Recipe

Serving: 24 | Prep: | Cook: 15mins | Ready in:

Ingredients

- 2 cups flour
- 1 cup cornstarch
- 1 cup powdered sugar

- 1/4 cup grated lemon zest
- 1 1/2 cups butter; softened
- colored sugars; optional

Direction

- Combine flour, corn starch, powdered sugar and lemon rind in a large bowl.
- With a large spoon, blend in butter, or blend in using electric mixer until a soft, smooth dough forms.
- Roll dough to 1/4" thickness.
- Cut into shapes with cookie cutters.
- Place on ungreased cookie sheets.
- Sprinkle with colored sugar.
- Bake at 300F for 15-20 minutes or until edges are lightly browned.
- Remove from sheet; cool completely.
- Makes about 4 dozen 2 1/2" cookies.

202. Lemon Squares Recipe

Serving: 0 | Prep: | Cook: 20mins | Ready in:

Ingredients

- 1 cup flour
- 1/2 cup sugar
- 3/4 cup margarine
- 1 1/2 cups graham wafer crumbs
- 1/4 cup coconut
- 2 tbls. milk
- 1/4 tsp. salt
- 1 tsp. baking powder
- 1 pkg. lemon pie filling

Direction

- Mix flour, sugar, graham crumbs, coconut, salt and baking powder together.
- Rub in margarine. Add milk and mix together.
- Spread half the mixture into a 9x13 pan.
- Prepare pie filling according to package directions.
- Spread over base.

- Spread other half of reserved mixture on top.
- Bake at 350 degrees for 15-20 minutes.

203. Lemon Tea Cookies Recipe

Serving: 3 | Prep: | Cook: 10mins | Ready in:

Ingredients

- cookies
- 1 cup butter or margarine, softened
- 1/3 cup powdered sugar
- 1 teaspoon vanilla
- 1 2/3 cups flour
- 1 tablespoon powdered sugar
- Filling
- 2/3 cup granulated sugar
- 3 teaspoons lemon peel, grated
- 3 tablespoons lemon juice
- 1 tablespoon butter or margarine
- 1 teaspoon cornstarch
- 1/4 teaspoon salt
- 1 egg, beaten

Direction

- In large bowl, Beat butter, 1/3 C powdered sugar, and vanilla with mixer on medium speed until well blended.
- Stir in flour until dough forms.
- Cover; refrigerate 30 minutes
- Heat oven to 350°F Shape dough into 1" balls.
- Place balls 2" apart. Press thumb into center of each ball to make indentation.
- Bake 8 to 10 minutes or until golden brown.
- Remove to cooling racks and cool completely, about 30 minutes.
- In 1 qt. saucepan, heat all filling ingredients over low heat about 25 minutes, stirring constantly, until smooth and thickened.
- Cool about 15 minutes.

- Fill each thumbprint with rounded 1/4 tsp. filling. Sprinkle 1 T powdered sugar over cookies.

204. Lemony Cheesecake Squares Recipe

Serving: 1 | Prep: | Cook: 45mins | Ready in:

Ingredients

- 2 C. vanilla wafer crumbs
- 1/4 C. sugar
- 1/2 C. butter melted
- 3 (8 oz) pkg. cream cheese softened
- 1 (14 oz) can Eagle Brand sweetened condensed milk (not evaporated milk)
- 3 eggs
- 1/2 C. lemon juice
- 3/4 C. strawberry preserves
- .

Direction

- Preheat oven to 375.
- Combine crumbs, sugar and butter; press firmly on bottom of 9x13 pan. Bake 8 minutes. Cool.
- Reduce oven temperature to 300.
- In large mixing bowl, beat cheese until fluffy. Gradually beat in condensed milk until smooth. Add eggs and lemon juice; mix well. Spread preserves evenly over prepared crust. Pour cheese mixture over preserves. Bake 45-50 minutes or until center is set. Cool. Chill. Refrigerate leftovers

205. Lime Lemon Twist Cookie Recipe

Serving: 24 | Prep: | Cook: 15mins | Ready in:

Ingredients

- 1 cup softened unsalted butter
- 3/4 cup sugar
- 1 egg
- 1 tsp pure lemon extract
- 1 -2 tsp lime rind
- 2 tbsp milk
- 1/4 tsp salt
- 2-1/2 cup flour
- 1/2 cup powdered sugar
- 2 tsp lemon juice

Direction

- Preheat oven to 350
- Grease cookie sheets
- In large bowl, beat butter & sugar till light and fluffy
- Add egg, lemon extract, lime rind & milk, and mix well
- Add 1 cup of flour at a time, blending well after each
- Form dough into ball and let sit 5 minutes
- Take a small walnut size of dough at a time and roll into 6" ropes
- (Use a little (and I mean little) flour to stop from sticking)
- Fold 6" rope in half and twist around each other
- Repeat till done
- Bake 12 minutes or till golden brown
- Topping:
- Mix 1/2 cup powdered sugar & lemon juice (add more lemon juice if too thick)
- Remove cookies from oven and immediately brush topping over hot cookies
- Cool on wire rack.

206. Lime Squares With Pistachio Graham Cracker Crust Recipe

Serving: 16 | Prep: | Cook: 12mins | Ready in:

Ingredients

- 4 tablespoons (1/2 stick) unsalted butter, melted and cooled, plus more for pan
- 2/3 cup shelled pistachios
- 1 cup (4 ounces) graham-cracker crumbs
- 1/4 cup sugar
- 1 tablespoons grated lime zest
- For the Filling:
- 2 large egg yolks
- 1 can (14 ounces) sweetened condensed milk
- 1/2 cup fresh lime juice

Direction

- Preheat oven to 350 degrees. Brush an 8-inch square baking dish with melted butter. Line bottom with parchment paper, leaving a 2-inch overhang on two sides.
- In a food processor, finely grind pistachios with graham-cracker crumbs, sugar, and zest. Blend in butter. Press mixture into bottom and 1 inch up sides of prepared pan. Bake until lightly browned, 8 to 12 minutes. Cool crust, 30 minutes.
- To make the filling: In a large bowl, whisk together egg yolks and condensed milk. Add lime juice; whisk until smooth. Pour filling into cooled crust; carefully spread to edges.
- Bake until set, about 15 minutes. Cool in pan on rack; then chill at least 1 hour before serving. Using parchment paper overhang, lift out of pan, and transfer to a cutting board. With a serrated knife, cut into 16 squares, wiping knife with a damp kitchen towel between each cut. To store in refrigerator, cover with plastic wrap.

---

207. Lotta Chocolate Mini Cookie Cups Recipe

Serving: 72 | Prep: | Cook: 16mins | Ready in:

Ingredients

- 3/4 cup butter or margarine
- 4 oz unsweetened baking chocolate
- 2 cups sugar
- 1 1/2 cups all-purpose flour
- 1/2 cup baking cocoa
- 2 teaspoons baking powder
- 1/2 teaspoon salt
- 4 eggs
- 1 1/2 cups semisweet chocolate chips
- 72 candied cherries, pecan or walnut halves, chocolate stars, etc..

Direction

- Heat oven to 350 degrees. Place mini paper baking cups in mini muffin pan cups (OR use mini foil muffin cups if you don't have mini muffin pans).
- In a 2-quart saucepan, melt butter and chocolate over low heat 6 to 10 minutes, stirring occasionally, until smooth (You can melt this in the microwave!); cool 20 minutes.
- In large bowl, beat melted chocolate, sugar, 1 cup flour, cocoa, baking powder, salt and eggs with mixer on medium speed about 2 minutes, scraping bowl occasionally, until well blended. Stir in remaining 1/2 cup flour and the chocolate chips. Drop dough by rounded teaspoons into prepared cups.
- Bake 15 to 17 minutes or until edges are slightly firm (centers should be slightly soft).
- Immediately top each with cherry, pecan or walnut half or chocolate, pressing slightly.

---

208. Lovers Lane Ultimate Fudge Cookie Recipe

Serving: 36 | Prep: | Cook: 10mins | Ready in:

Ingredients

- 6 tablespoons unsalted butter
- 1-12 ounce package semisweet chocolate chips
- 1-14 ounce can sweetened condensed milk
- 1 cup all-purpose flour

- 1 cups chopped pecans

Direction

- In heavy saucepan, combine butter, chocolate chips and milk
- Cook over low heat, stirring often, until chocolate is melted and mixture is smooth
- Stir flour and pecans into chocolate mixture
- Drop dough by teaspoonful onto lightly greased cookie sheet
- Bake at 300 degrees for about 10 minutes, or until light glaze forms on cookies
- Cookies will not appear done, but please do not over bake
- Cool on wire rack

209. Low Country Cookies Recipe Courtesy Paula Deen Recipe

Serving: 12 | Prep: | Cook: | Ready in:

Ingredients

- Filling:
- 1 (16-ounce) box graham crackers
- 12 tablespoons (1 1/2 sticks) butter
- 1 cup sugar
- 1 egg
- 1/2 cup milk
- 1 cup chopped pecans
- 1 cup or 3 (1/2-ounce) cans shredded coconut
- Topping:
- 2 cups powdered sugar
- 1 teaspoon vanilla
- 4 tablespoons (1/2 stick) butter
- 3 tablespoons milk

Direction

- For the filling: Line a 13 by 9-inch pan with whole graham crackers. Melt the butter in saucepan and add sugar. Beat the egg and milk together; add to butter mixture. Bring to a

boil, stirring constantly. Remove from heat. Add the nuts, coconut, and 1 cup graham cracker crumbs. Pour over the crackers in the pan. Cover with another layer of whole graham crackers.
- For the topping: Beat all the ingredients together and spread over top layer of crackers.
- Chill. Cut into squares.

210. Low Fat Lemon Raspberry Cookies Recipe

Serving: 24 | Prep: | Cook: 12mins | Ready in:

Ingredients

- 1/2 cup I Can't Believe It's Not Butter light
- 3/4 cup plus 1/4 cup sugar, divided
- 1 tspn finely shredded lemon peel
- 1 tspn baking powder
- 1/4 tspn baking soda
- 1 egg
- 1/3 cup fat-free skim milk
- 2 tspns plus 2 Tablespoons lemon juice, divided
- 1 3/4 cup all-purpose flour
- 1/2 cup raspberry jam/jelly/preserves

Direction

- 1) In large mixing bowl, beat the margarine with an electric mixer for 30 seconds. Add 3/4 cup sugar, lemon zest, baking powder, and baking soda. Beat until combined.
- 2) Beat in egg, milk, and 2 tsps. lemon juice
- 3) Beat in the flour, until combined.
- 4) Drop dough by rounded teaspoons on ungreased cookie sheet, and bake at 350 for 7 minutes (half-way point), pull out the cookies and use the back of a metal teaspoon to make a "thumbprint" to each cookie. If cookie sticks to spoon, use a little flour on the back of spoon. In each thumbprint place 1 tsp. raspberry jelly/jam, return back to oven to continue to bake for 7 minutes.

5) After cookies are done, mix together 2 tbsp. fresh lemon juice with 1/4 cup sugar and brush on all cookie tops.

211. Lowfat Raisin Oatmeal Cookies Recipe

Serving: 40 | Prep: | Cook: 11mins | Ready in:

Ingredients

- 1 cup wholewheat flour
- 1 tsp. baking powder
- 1 tsp. cinnamon
- 1/ tsp. baking soda
- 1/ tsp, salt
- 1 cup packed bown sugar{May use light brown sugar}
- 1/4 cup fat free vanilla yogurt
- 2 tbls. corn oil
- 1 large egg
- 1 tsp, vanilla
- 1 1/2c ups old fashion rolled oats

Direction

- Heat oven to 350 degrees cover cookie sheets with parchment paper
- Combined flour, baking powder, cinnamon and baking soda and salt into small bowl\Combined brown sugar yogurt oil egg and vanilla in large bowl add flour mixture stir l well.
- Stir in oats and raisins drop by rounded teaspoons 2 inches apart on cookie sheets Bake 10-12 minutes till lightly brown {DO NOT OVERBAKE} After done slide cookies onto parchment paper to cool on counter top

212. Lunch Lady Butter Sugar Cookies Recipe

Serving: 24 | Prep: | Cook: 10mins | Ready in:

Ingredients

- 2 sticks butter(1 cup)
- 2/3 cup sugar
- 2 cups plus 2 tablespoons all-purpose flour
- 2 teaspoons vanilla

Direction

- Preheat oven to 350 degrees F
- Cream butter & sugar until light & fluffy.
- Add vanilla
- Mix flour a little bit at a time, mixing well
- Roll dough into balls
- Flatten on ungreased cookie sheet
- Bake until golden brown
- Approximately 8 - 10 minutes ...watching carefully
- Enjoy!
- **
- Be flexible with changing your plans
- **

213. Luscious Layer Bars Recipe

Serving: 36 | Prep: | Cook: 45mins | Ready in:

Ingredients

- 1 pouch chocolate chip cookie mix (Betty Crocker)
- 1/2 cup butter or margarine, softened
- 1 egg
- 1 cup butterscotch chips
- 1 cup of milk chocolate chips or semi-sweet chocolate chips
- 1 cup of flaked coconut

- 1 cup of chopped walnuts
- 1 can (140z) sweetened condensed milk (not evaporated)

Direction

- Heat oven to 350 Spray bottom of 13x9-inch pan with cooking spray (You can skip the spray and line the pan with foil to make cleanup and bar removal easier)
- In large bowl, stir cookie mix, butter and egg until soft dough forms. Press dough in bottom of pan using floured fingers
- Bake 15 minutes. Sprinkle with butterscotch chips, chocolate chips, coconut & walnuts. Drizzle evenly with condensed milk.
- Bake 30 to 35 minutes or until light golden brown. Cool completely, about 2 hours. For bars, cut into 9 rows by 4 rows.

214. Luscious Lime Angel Squares Recipe

Serving: 15 | Prep: | Cook: 5mins | Ready in:

Ingredients

- 1 package sugar free lime gelatin (.3 ounce)
- 1 cup boiling water
- 1 prepared angel food cake, cut into 1 inch cubes
- 1 package reduced fat cream cheese cubed
- 1/2 cup sugar
- 2 teaspoons lemon juice
- 1 1/2 teaspoons lemon zest
- 1 carton reduced fat whipped topping, thawed, divided (8 ounces)

Direction

- In a bowl, dissolve gelatine in boiling water,
- Refrigerate until mixture just begins to thickens, about 35 minutes.
- Place cake cubes in a 13 x 9 x 2 inch dish coated with non-stick cooking spray; set aside.

- In a small mixing bowl, beat cream cheese until smooth.
- Beat in sugar, lemon juice and zest.
- Add gelatine mixture; beat until combined.
- Fold in 1 1/2 cups whipped topping.
- Spread over cake, covering completely.
- Refrigerate for at least 2 hours or until firm.
- Cut into squares; top with remaining whipped topping.

215. Macaroon Kisses Recipe

Serving: 48 | Prep: | Cook: 15mins | Ready in:

Ingredients

- 1 (14-ounce) can Eagle Brand sweetened condensed milk
- (NOT evaporated milk)
- 2 teaspoons vanilla extract
- 1 to 1 1/2 teaspoons almond extract
- 2 (7-ounce) packages flaked coconut (5 1/3 cups)
- 48 solid milk chocolate candy kisses, stars or drops

Direction

- 1. Preheat oven to 325. Line baking sheets with foil; grease and flour foil. Set aside.
- 2. In large bowl, combine Eagle Brand, vanilla and almond extract. Stir in coconut.
- Drop by rounded teaspoonful onto foil-lined sheets; with spoon, slightly flatten each mound.
- 3. Bake 15 to 17 minutes or until golden. Remove from oven. Immediately press candy kiss, star or drop in center of each macaroon.
- Remove from baking sheets; cool on wire racks.
- Store loosely covered at room temperature

216.   Mads' Delicious Moist Cookies Recipe

Serving: 0 | Prep: | Cook: 7mins | Ready in:

Ingredients

- 1 C all purpose flour
- 1 C oats
- 3/4 t baking powder
- 1/4 t baking soda
- 1/2 C cane sugar
- 3/4 C vanilla soy yogurt
- 1 vanilla soy milk
- 1 T butter

Direction

- 1. Prepare yourself a glass of wine. Enjoy throughout baking.
- 2. In large bowl, mix dry ingredients together.
- 3. While stirring in between additions, add in yogurt, milk, and softened butter.
- 4. Mix well while oven preheats.
- 5. Lightly oil 2 cookie sheets. Cookie mixture will not be very thick. Make sure you leave room for the cookies to expand while in the oven- they'll get big!
- 6. After about 7 minutes peek into the oven to see if they appear done. You can wait until the edges brown if preferred; I like mine chewy so I took them out just before.
- 7. Eat, share & enjoy! :D

217.   Maricas Dreamy Chocolate Peanutty Crumple Square Recipe

Serving: 8 | Prep: | Cook: 25mins | Ready in:

Ingredients

- 1/2 cup butter or margarine
- 1 cup all - purpose flour
- 3/4 cup instant oats (uncooked)

- 1/3 cup brown sugar
- 1/2 tsp baking soda
- 1/2 tsp vanilla extract
- 4 (2.23 - ounce) Snickers bars (cut into 8 slices each)

Direction

- Preheat oven to 350 degrees oven.
- Grease the bottom of an 8-inch square pan.
- In a large saucepan melt the butter or margarine. Remove the pan from the heat and stir in the flour, oats, brown sugar, baking soda and vanilla. Blend until crumbly. Press 2/3 of the mixture into the prepared pan. Arrange the Snickers bar slices in the pan, about 1/2-inch from the edge of the pan. Finely crumble the remaining mixture over the sliced Snickers bars.
- Bake for 25 minutes or until edges are golden brown. Cool in the pan on a cooling rack. Cut into bars or squares to serve. Makes 24 bars

218.   Merry Berry Cheese Bars Recipe

Serving: 15 | Prep: | Cook: 45mins | Ready in:

Ingredients

- 2 cups unsifted flour
- 11/2 cups oats
- 3/4 cup + 1tbsp firmly packed brown sugar
- 1 cup butter, softened
- 8 oz. cream cheese, softened
- 14 oz. sweetened condensed milk
- 1/4 cup ReaLemon lemon juice from concentrate
- 16 oz. can whole berry cranberry sauce
- 2tbsp corn starch

Direction

- Preheat oven to 350

- With mixer, beat flour, oats, 3/4 cup sugar, & butter until crumbly.
- Set aside 1/2 cups mixture; press remaining mixture on bottom of greased 13+9 baking pan.
- Bake 15 minutes or until lightly browned
- With Mixer, beat cheese until fluffy.
- Gradually beat in sweetened condensed milk until smooth
- Stir in lemon.
- Spread over baked crust.
- Combine cranberry sauce, corn starch and remaining 1tbsp sugar.
- Spoon over cheese layer.
- Top with reserved crumb mixture
- Bake 45 minutes or until golden brown.
- Cool & cut into bars
- Refrigerate leftovers.

219. Mexican Aniseed Cookies Recipe

Serving: 24 | Prep: | Cook: 20mins | Ready in:

Ingredients

- 1-1/2 cups all purpose flour
- 1 teaspoon baking powder
- 1/8 teaspoon salt
- 1/2 cup unsalted butter
- 1/2 cup sugar
- 1 egg
- 1 teaspoon whole aniseed
- 1 tablespoon brandy
- 1/4 cup sugar mixed with 1/2 teaspoon cinnamon

Direction

- Sift together flour, baking powder and salt then set aside.
- Beat butter with sugar until soft and fluffy.
- Add egg, aniseed and brandy and beat until incorporated.

- Fold in dry ingredients until just blended to a dough then chill 30 minutes.
- Preheat oven to 350 then grease 2 baking sheets.
- On a lightly floured surface roll out chilled dough to 1/8" thick.
- With floured cutter or knife cut out cookies into squares.
- Place on prepared baking sheets and sprinkle lightly with cinnamon sugar.
- Bake for 10 minutes until just barely golden.
- Cool on sheets for 5 minutes before transferring to wire rack to cool completely.

220. Mexican Cookies Recipe

Serving: 2 | Prep: | Cook: 25mins | Ready in:

Ingredients

- 1 cup butter
- 1 cup powdered sugar divided
- 1 1/2 Tsp. vanilla
- 2 cups sifted flour
- 1/2 cup chopped nuts {your choice}

Direction

- Preheat oven 325
- In a bowl cream butter 3/4 cup powdered sugar and vanilla
- Add flour and nuts gradually mix until blended
- Form into 1-inch Balls
- Bake for 25 minutes
- Roll immediately in remaining 1/4 cup sugar
- Allow to cool and roll in sugar again.
- Given to me by a friend {have made them delicious cookies}

221. Millionaires Shortbread Recipe

Serving: 18 | Prep: | Cook: 30mins | Ready in:

Ingredients

- SHORTBREAD:
- 2 sticks butter, cut into small pieces, plus more for preparing pans
- 2 cups all purpose flour, plus more for pans
- 2/3 cup sugar
- 1/2 t salt
- caramel LAYER:
- 2 (14oz) cans sweetened condensed milk
- 2 T butter
- chocolate TOPPING:
- 3/4 pound good-quality milk chocolate

Direction

- Preheat oven to 350 degrees
- Butter 2 (8in) square nonstick pans and coat with flour
- Place flour, sugar and salt in food processor and pulse once
- Add butter and pulse until mixture resembles peas
- Press the shortbread mixture into pans and bake until golden brown around the edges, about 20 minutes
- Remove from the oven and let cool completely
- Caramel Layer:
- In a heavy bottomed saucepan over medium low heat, combine the condensed milk and 2 T of butter
- Slowly bring the mixture to a boil, stirring continuously
- Continue stirring until mixture becomes thick and amber in color, about 15 minutes
- Pour over the cooked shortbread and spread evenly
- Cool to room temperature
- Chocolate Topping:
- In a glass bowl, melt chocolate in the microwave about 2 minutes, stirring every 30 seconds or so until melted
- Pour over the cooled caramel

222. Mint Chcoalte Chip Cookies Im Awesome Recipe

Serving: 8 | Prep: | Cook: 10mins | Ready in:

Ingredients

- 2 3/4 cups all-purpose flour
- 1 teaspoon baking soda
- 1 teaspoon salt
- 1 cup (2 sticks, 1/2 pound) butter, softened
- 3/4 cup granulated [white] sugar
- 3/4 cup packed brown sugar
- 1 teaspoon peppermint extract
- 2 eggs
- 2 cups (12-ounce package) NESTLE TOLL HOUSE Semi-sweet chocolate Morsels

Direction

- PREHEAT THE OVEN AT 375 DEGREES F
- Start with the butter (or Crisco) with the sugar and mix until well-blended. Once done with that, add everything except for the flour and 'chips.
- If you want fluffy cookies use a blender, if you want chewy cookies mix with a fork, by hand, not that hard.
- The next step is to add the flour a little at a time, you don't want to whip it out of the bowl, or get tired mixing.
- Lastly add the chocolate chips and fold them in.
- If you haven't preheated the oven, you are one poor sucker. Roll the cookies into balls as big as you want, and put into the oven for ten minutes only. Don't go over that time or they'll be over-cooked.

223. Mmmolasses Cookies Recipe

Serving: 36 | Prep: | Cook: 12mins | Ready in:

Ingredients

- 1 cup molasses
- 1 egg
- 1 Tbsp. baking soda
- 2 tsp ginger
- 1 Tbsp. white vinegar
- 1 tsp. cloves
- 1 cup shortening or 1/2 cup shortening and 1/2 cup butter/margarine
- 1 tsp. salt
- 1 cup brown sugar
- 4 cups all-purpose flour

Direction

- In a large saucepan, bring molasses to a boil.
- Add soda and vinegar.
- Note: Now, we all know the chemical reaction that occurs when we combine baking soda and vinegar. So, be prepared for some bubbling up!!!
- Blend well and cool.
- Add shortening, brown sugar, egg and dry ingredients sifted together.
- Roll out (I scooped by the Tbsp.) and bake in a moderate 350 degree oven for 10-12 minutes.
- These may be rolled in cling wrap and stored in the refrigerator until needed at which time they are sliced and baked.

224. Mocha Frosted Drops Recipe

Serving: 25 | Prep: | Cook: 10mins | Ready in:

Ingredients

- 1/2 cup shortening
- 2 1-oune squares unsweetened chocolate

- 1 cup brown sugar
- 1 egg
- 1 tsp vanlla
- 1/2 cup buttermilk
- 1 1/2 cups sifted all-pupose flour
- 1/2 tsp baking powder
- 1/2 tsp baking soda
- 1/4 tsp salt
- 1/2 cup chopped walnuts
- 1 6-ounce package(1 cup) semi-sweet chocolate chips
- Mocha frosting

Direction

- Melt shortening and unsweetened chocolate squares together in sauce pan
- Let cool 10 minutes
- Stir in brown sugar
- Beat in the egg, vanilla, and buttermilk
- Sift together dry ingredients and add to chocolate mixture
- Stir in nuts and chocolate pieces
- Drop from teaspoon on greased cookie sheet
- Bake at 375 degrees for 10 minutes
- Remove from pan and cool
- Frost with mocha frosting
- Top with walnut (optional)
- Makes 3 1/2 dozen cookies

225. Mocha Sugar Cookies Recipe

Serving: 24 | Prep: | Cook: 15mins | Ready in:

Ingredients

- 1/3 cup vegetable shortening
- 1/2 cup brown sugar packed
- 1/2 cup granulated sugar
- 1 egg
- 1-1/2 teaspoons vanilla extract
- 1 tablespoon milk
- 2 tablespoons instant coffee powder

- 2 cups flour
- 1/2 teaspoon salt
- 1/2 teaspoon baking soda
- 1/4 teaspoon baking powder
- 2 ounce chocolate bar coarsely grated

Direction

- In mixing bowl cream together shortening and sugars then add egg and vanilla.
- Heat milk and stir in instant coffee and add to creamed mixture and mix well.
- Sift flour, salt, baking soda and baking powder and add to creamed mixture and mix well.
- Roll mixture into 1" balls and place on ungreased baking sheets well-spaced apart.
- Press out cookie with bottom of lightly buttered glass dipped in sugar or press with fork.
- Sprinkle lightly with grated chocolate then bake at 375 for 10 minutes.
- Cool slightly before removing to wire racks and cool completely.

226. Molasses Sugar Cookies Recipe

Serving: 24 | Prep: | Cook: 10mins |Ready in:

Ingredients

- 2-1/4 cups flour
- 2 teaspoons baking soda
- 1 teaspoon cinnamon
- 1/2 teaspoon cloves
- 1/2 teaspoon ginger
- 1/2 teaspoon salt
- 3/4 cups oleo
- 1 cup sugar
- 1/4 cup molasses
- 1 egg
- sugar in bowl for coating balls

Direction

- Combine flour, baking soda, cinnamon, cloves, ginger and salt in a bowl.
- Melt oleo over low heat and cool.
- Beat in 1 cup of sugar, the molasses, and egg.
- Add dry ingredients; mix well.
- Shape dough into balls, using a rounded teaspoon for each
- Roll balls in sugar and place on lightly greased baking sheet
- Bake at 375 degrees for about 10 minutes

227. Molasses With Raisins Cookies Recipe

Serving: 44 | Prep: | Cook: 27mins |Ready in:

Ingredients

- 3-1/4 cups all-purpose flour
- 1 teaspoon baking soda
- 1/4 teaspoon salt
- 2 teaspoons ground cinnamon
- 1 teaspoon ground ginger
- 1/2 teaspoon allspice
- 1 cup (packed) dark brown sugar
- 2 sticks (1 cup) salted butter, softened
- 3/4 cup molasses
- 1 large egg
- 1-1/2 cups raisins or approximately 6 ounces which have been soaked for 10 minutes in boiling water with a splash of Irish whiskey ;-) then drained well. Don't throw the liquid away, save it for another recipe!!!
- Icing:
- 1 (8 ounce) packages cream cheese, softened
- 1/2 stick (1/4 cup) salted butter, softened
- 1 cups powdered sugar
- 1/2 teaspoon vanilla extract

Direction

- In a medium bowl, whisk together flour, baking soda, salt cinnamon, ginger, and allspice; set aside.

- In a large bowl, with an electric mixer, beat together butter and sugar to form a grainy paste.
- Add molasses and egg, scraping down side as needed, beat until light and fluffy.
- Add flour mixture and raisins, and blend at low speed until just combined.
- Divide dough in half and form into logs 1-1/2-inch in diameter.
- Wrap both logs with wax paper and chill in refrigerator for 2 hours.
- After dough has chilled, preheat oven to 300 degrees F.
- Remove wax paper and slice dough into 1/2-inch size pieces.
- Place pieces flat side down 1-1/2 inches apart on an ungreased cookie sheet.
- Bake for 25-27 minutes until cookies are set.
- Transfer cookies immediately to cooling surface.
- Icing:
- In a large bowl, cream together the cream cheese and butter with an electric mixer.
- Mix in vanilla extract.
- Gradually stir in powdered sugar, until well blended. Store in refrigerator after use.
- Using a small spoon or knife lightly spread a small circle of icing onto centre of each cookie.
- This recipe makes approximately 44 cookies.

---

228. Monster Cookie Jar Mix Recipe

Serving: 24 | Prep: | Cook: 1hours | Ready in:

Ingredients

- Mix
- 1/2 cup vanilla sugar (or regular)
- 1 tsp baking soda
- 1/2 tsp sea salt
- 2 1/4 cups rolled oats

- 1 cup assorted candy, nuts and fruit (I used a box of Smarties and 2/3 cup of Chocolicious Snack Mix from Bulk Barn)
- 1/2 cup packed dark brown sugar
- 1/4 cup miniature chocolate chips
- To prepare:
- 3/4 cup smooth peanut butter (not natural)
- 2 tbsp salted butter, softened
- 2 eggs
- 1 tsp vanilla (if you didn't use vanilla sugar in the mix)

Direction

- Mix
- Mix together the vanilla sugar, baking soda and salt in a small dish and place in the bottom of a 1-quart jar.
- Layer with the oats, then the candy, brown sugar and chocolate chips.
- Seal the jar and attach directions:
- To prepare:
- Mix together the peanut butter, butter, eggs and vanilla (if using) until well combined.
- Add the jar mix and stir well to combine.
- Refrigerate 30 minutes.
- Preheat the oven to 350F and line three cookie sheets with parchment.
- Form 2" balls and place no less than 2" apart on the sheets.
- Bake 14 minutes.
- Cool on the sheets for 10 minutes, then remove to a wire rack and cool completely.

---

229. Monster Mash Cookies Recipe

Serving: 36 | Prep: | Cook: 1hours | Ready in:

Ingredients

- ⅔ cup granulated sugar
- ⅔ cup brown sugar, packed
- 1 tsp kosher salt

- ¾ cup non-hydrogenated shortening
- ¼ cup ricotta (I used homemade Richer Ricotta)
- 2 eggs
- 1 tbsp vanilla
- 2 tbsp corn syrup
- 2 ½ cups white whole wheat flour
- 1 tsp baking soda
- ¼ tsp nutmeg
- 150g (two "super-size" boxes) Smarties chocolate candy (or M&M's)
- ⅓ cup miniature chocolate chips
- ½ cup sprinkles, for crusting

Direction

- Preheat oven to 375F
- Beat together the sugars, salt, shortening and ricotta until light and fluffy.
- Beat in the eggs, vanilla and corn syrup until well blended.
- Add the flour, baking soda and nutmeg, followed by the Smarties and chocolate chips.
- Pour sprinkles into a shallow dish. Scoop balls of dough and lightly press the tops in the sprinkles to crust.
- Bake for 13 minutes.
- Cool completely on sheets.

230.   Moose Poop Cookies Recipe

Serving: 5 | Prep: | Cook: 20mins | Ready in:

Ingredients

- 2 sticks of butter
- 3/4 cup brown sugar
- 3/4 cup white sugar
- 2 eggs
- 1 tsp vanilla
- 2 cups flour
- 1/2 tsp salt
- 1 tsp baking soda

- 3 cups oatmeal
- 1 cup chopped walnuts
- 2 cups chocolate chips

Direction

- Mix all together.
- Drop by 1/4 cup portions on a greased cookie sheet.
- Bake at 325 degrees for 20 minutes.

231.   Mudhen Bars Recipe

Serving: 32 | Prep: | Cook: 40mins | Ready in:

Ingredients

- 1/2 cup shortening
- 1 cup sugar
- 3 eggs, 1 whole and 2 separated
- 1 1/2 cups flour
- 1 tsp. baking powder
- 1/4 tsp.salt
- 1 cup chopped walnuts
- 1 cup chocolate chips
- 1 cup coconut
- 1 cup mini marshmallows
- 1 cup brown sugar, packed

Direction

- Preheat oven to 350.
- Cream shortening and sugar.
- Beat in 1 whole egg and 2 yolks.
- Stir in flour, baking powder and salt.
- Spread into a 9x13 pan.
- Sprinkle with nuts, chips, coconut and marshmallows.
- Beat the 2 egg whites until stiff.
- Fold in the brown sugar and spread over cake.
- Bake 30-40 minutes.

232. New Generation Apple Squares Recipe

Serving: 12 | Prep: | Cook: 1hours | Ready in:

Ingredients

- 1 cup rolled oats (not instant)
- 1/2 cup spelt flakes
- 1 1/2 cups oat flour (or whole wheat flour)
- 1/4 tsp baking soda
- 1/4 tsp salt
- 2/3 cup dark brown sugar
- 3.5 oz salted butter
- 2 tbsp low fat milk
- 3 cups Butterscotch Apple Pie Filling or canned apple pie filling + 2 tbsp butterscotch sauce

Direction

- Preheat oven to 375F.
- In a large bowl combine the oats, spelt flakes, flour, baking soda, salt and brown sugar.
- Cut in the butter until it is the size of peas, then add the milk and mix until crumbly but "packable".
- Press half of the mixture into the bottom of a 9" square pan.
- Evenly spread the Butterscotch Apple Pie Filling overtop and press the remaining crumble on gently.
- Place pan on a cookie sheet and bake for 45 minutes.
- Cool at least 15 minutes before cutting.

233. Nighty Nights Recipe

Serving: 24 | Prep: | Cook: 480mins | Ready in:

Ingredients

- I put 480 minutes because these bake overnight...
- 2 egg whites

- pinch of salt
- 3/4 c. sugar
- 1 tsp. vanilla
- 1/2 c. chopped pecans
- 3/4 c. chocolate chips

Direction

- Preheat oven to 350
- Beat egg whites and pinch of salt until fluffy
- Add the sugar slowly, 1 tbsp. at a time, scraping bowl often, until all the sugar is added, should be getting stiffer
- Beat in the vanilla
- Fold in the nuts and chocolate chips, gently
- Drop by teaspoonful onto cookie sheets lined with foil
- Put in the preheated oven, then TURN THE OVEN OFF!!!
- Don't open the door!!!
- The cookies will be ready when you wake up in the morning....

234. Nitey Nite Cookies Recipe

Serving: 24 | Prep: | Cook: | Ready in:

Ingredients

- 2 egg whites
- 2/3 cup sugar
- 1 cup chopped nuts
- 1 cup chocolate chips

Direction

- Preheat oven to 350 degrees. Beat eggs until fluffy, and gradually add sugar. Beat until stiff. Stir in nuts and chocolate chips. Drop on foil lined pan. Put in oven, close door, turn oven off. DON'T OPEN UNTIL MORNING!!

235. No Bake Cookies Recipe

Serving: 3 | Prep: | Cook: 1mins | Ready in:

Ingredients

- 2 1/2 cups granulated sugar
- 2 T unsweetened cocoa
- 1/2 cup butter
- 1/2 cup milk
- 1 t vanilla
- 1/2 cup creamy peanut butter
- 3 cups quick cooking rolled oats, uncooked

Direction

- In a medium saucepan, combine sugar, cocoa, butter and milk.
- Bring to a boil; boil for 1 minute. (Use a timer - don't overcook.)
- Stir in vanilla, peanut butter and oats; mix thoroughly.
- Drop by spoonfuls onto waxed paper.
- Let cool.

236. No Bake Fudge Cookies Recipe

Serving: 12 | Prep: | Cook: 5mins | Ready in:

Ingredients

- Ingredients:
- 2 cups of sugar or sugar substitute
- ½ cup cocoa
- ½ cup milk
- ½ cup butter or margarine
- Other Ingredients:
- 3 cups oats
- 1 cup chopped walnuts
- ½ cup raisins
- 1 teas. vanilla
- Coating:
- Optional: powdered sugar

Direction

- Combine all the ingredients (except the other ingredients and coating) in a 4 quart pan on stove stir on medium heat until it is a rolling boil. Boil for 4 minutes.
- In the pan add all the other ingredients stir. On a foil line baking sheet drop teaspoonfuls of mixture on foil. Let set. After it is firm add coating.

237. No Bake Chocolate Oat Bars Recipe

Serving: 12 | Prep: | Cook: 3mins | Ready in:

Ingredients

- 1 cup butter
- ½ cup brown sugar, packed
- 1 teasp vanilla
- 3 cups Uncooked quick oats
- 1 cup chocolate chips
- ½ cup peanut butter

Direction

- Grease 9" square baking pan.
- Melt butter in large sauce pan over medium heat. Add sugar and vanilla. Stir in oats and cook over low heat two to three minutes or until well blended.
- Press 1/2 mixture into pan.
- Melt chocolate chips, and peanut butter and pour over mixture in pan.
- Crumble remaining mixture over top of chocolate and press in gently. Cover and refrigerate two to three hours or until firm.
- Bring to room temperature before cutting into squares.

238. Noci Di Burro Butter Nuts Recipe

Serving: 50 | Prep: | Cook: 20mins | Ready in:

Ingredients

- ½ lb butter, softened
- 1/3 cup confectioners' sugar
- 1 teaspoon vanilla
- 2 cups flour
- 1 cup hazelnuts, chopped
- confectioner's sugar for coating

Direction

- Preheat oven to 350.
- Using an electric mixer, cream butter, confectioners' sugar, and vanilla until well blended.
- Add flour and hazelnuts on low speed.
- Roll dough into ½ inch balls and place on parchment lined cookie sheets, spacing them about 2 inches apart.
- Bake 15 to 20 minutes, or until lightly browned.
- Remove the cookie sheet from the oven.
- While cookies are hot, roll in confectioner's sugar to coat.
- Store in an airtight container. Re-roll in sugar before serving.
- Yields 50 cookies.

239. Northern Gold Energy Bar Recipe

Serving: 24 | Prep: | Cook: 10mins | Ready in:

Ingredients

- 280g (small bag) marshmallows
- 3 tbsp (30g) butter
- 26g pine nuts
- 425g (6 cups) whole crispy puffed rice
- 90g (3/4 cups) golden raisins
- 14g (1 scoop) Pierce Lean Whey powder

Direction

- Line a small baking tray with wax paper.
- Melt butter in a large glass bowl in microwave, 1 minute on defrost
- Add marshmallows and stir to coat. Microwave on low for about two minutes or until marshmallows start to melt.
- Quickly stir in whey protein with a silicon spatula and then add the rest of the ingredients.
- Evenly coat the puffed rice with the cooling marshmallows with oiled hands.
- Spread out the mixture on to the baking tray.
- Cut in to squares.

240. Norwegian Serinakaker Or Serina Cookies Recipe

Serving: 26 | Prep: | Cook: 12mins | Ready in:

Ingredients

- 1 cup cold butter (not margarine)
- 2 cups all-purpose flour
- 1/2 teaspoon baking powder
- 2 eggs
- 3/4 cup granulated sugar
- 1 tablespoon vanilla sugar
- (or substitute 1 tablespoon sugar and 1 tsp. vanilla)
- 1 cup chopped almonds

Direction

- Cut butter into small pieces in the mixer's bowl, stir in the flour and baking powder.
- Blend with an electric mixer on medium speed until well blended.
- Add one egg, reserving the other, to the mixture, then blend at medium speed for 1 minute.

- Add the sugar and vanilla sugar while continuing to blend at medium speed, about one more minute.
- Refrigerate the dough in a covered container for two or three hours.
- Beat the other egg.
- Roll the dough into small balls, about 3/4" round, and place on ungreased cookie sheet 2" apart.
- Flatten each ball slightly with either a fork or a cookie stamp.
- Brush the top of the cookies with egg and sprinkle some chopped almonds on top.
- Bake at 375°F for 8-12 minutes or until golden brown.
- Cool the cookies.
- Makes approximately 26.
- Note: Vanilla sugar is available at many European Delicatessen's specializing in German, Swedish and other European foods.

241.   Nut Macaroons Recipe

Serving: 40 | Prep: | Cook: 5mins | Ready in:

Ingredients

- 3 egg whites
- 1/4 teaspoon cream of tartar
- 1 cup sugar
- 1 tablespoon all-purpose flour
- 2 cups finely chopped hickory nuts or pecans
- Desired candied fruit pieces

Direction

- 1. Beat egg whites and cream of tartar in mixing bowl with an electric mixer until soft peaks form (tips bend over). Gradually add sugar, beating at high speed until stiff peaks form. Fold in flour and nuts.
- 2. Drop by rounded teaspoons onto a parchment-paper-lined cookie sheet. Bake in a 400-degree F oven for 5 to 7 minutes or until lightly browned. Cool 1 to 2 minutes; press a

piece of candied fruit into the top of each cookie. Remove and cool on wire rack.
- Makes about 40 cookies.

242.   Nutella Meringues Recipe

Serving: 25 | Prep: | Cook: 190mins | Ready in:

Ingredients

- 3 egg whites
- pinch cream of tartar
- pinch of salt (I used vanilla salt)
- 1/3 cup vanilla (or regular granulated) sugar
- 1/4 cup nutella, warmed until runny

Direction

- Preheat the oven to 300F and set one oven rack in the bottom third of your oven and one in the upper third of your oven.
- Line two baking sheets with parchment paper and set aside.
- Beat egg whites, cream of tartar and salt until soft peaks form.
- Increase the speed to high and begin adding the sugar a few spoonfuls at a time.
- Continue beating to stiff peaks.
- Remove the bowl from the mixer and add all the Nutella.
- With a rubber spatula, gently fold the Nutella into the meringue three or four times until just swirled. Don't over mix - this will deflate the meringue.
- Place in the oven for 10 minutes. After 10 minutes, immediately lower the heat to 200 F and rotate the trays. Bake for an hour.
- If they are completely dried by then, turn the oven off and leave the meringues in the oven for a few hours to cool with the oven.
- If the meringues still look a bit "wet", then continue baking for another 20 minutes or so.

243.   Nutella Sandwich Cookies Recipe

Serving: 0 | Prep: | Cook: 30mins | Ready in:

Ingredients

- 1/2 cup unsalted butter, softened
- 1/2 cup nutella
- 3/4 cup granulated sugar
- 1 egg
- 1 teaspoon pure vanilla extract
- 3 cups flour
- 1 teaspoon baking powder
- 1/2 teaspoon sea salt
- Approx. 1/4 cup heavy cream

Direction

- 1. Preheat the oven to 350°F. Lightly grease a baking sheet and set aside.
- 2. Beat together the butter, Nutella, and sugar until light and fluffy. Add the egg and vanilla and beat until well incorporated.
- 3. In a separate mixing bowl, whisk together the flour, baking powder, and sea salt. Gradually add the dry ingredients to the creamed mixture, mixing on low speed, until the dough begins to come together. If the dough seems dry and crumbly, add a small amount of heavy cream until the dough comes together.
- 4. Transfer the dough to a lightly floured surface and roll it out to about 1/4-inch thickness. Use a cookie cutter to cut shapes out of the dough and transfer them to the prepared baking sheet.
- 5. Bake the cookies for about 12 minutes. Let them cool for a few minutes on the baking sheets, and then transfer to wire racks to cool completely.
- 6. Frost cookies or spread Nutella on one cookie and cover it with another. Enjoy!

244.   Nutty Chocolate Caramel Delights Recipe

Serving: 18 | Prep: | Cook: 20mins | Ready in:

Ingredients

- 1 package German chocolate cake mix
- 1 cup chopped pecans
- 1/3 cup plus 1/2 cup evaporated milk divided
- 3/4 cup butter melted
- 14 ounce package vanilla caramels unwrapped
- 1 cup semisweet chocolate morsels

Direction

- In large mixing bowl combine dry cake mix, pecans, 1/3 cup evaporated milk and melted butter.
- Press half the batter into bottom of a greased rectangular glass baking dish.
- Bake in a preheated 350 oven for 8 minutes.
- In top of a double boiler over simmering water melt caramels with remaining milk.
- When caramel mixture is well blended pour over baked layer then cover with chocolate morsels.
- Pour remaining batter on top of morsels then return to preheated 350 oven and bake 10 minutes.
- Let cool before cutting into squares.

245.   OATMEAL RAISIN COOKIES Recipe

Serving: 24 | Prep: | Cook: 10mins | Ready in:

Ingredients

- 1 cup all-purpose flour
- 1 teaspoon cinnamon
- 1 teaspoon salt
- 1/2 teaspoon baking soda
- 3/4 cup butter-flavored shortening
- 1 cup packed brown sugar

- 1/2 cup granulated sugar
- 1 egg
- 1/4 cup water
- 2 teaspoons vanilla extract
- 1 cup raisins
- 1 cup chopped nuts (optional)
- 1/2 cup wheat germ (optional)
- 3 cups old fashioned rolled oats or quick cooking oats

Direction

- Heat oven to 350 degrees.
- In a medium bowl, combine flour, cinnamon, salt, and baking soda; set aside.
- In a large bowl, cream together shortening, brown sugar, and granulated sugar. Stir in egg, water, and vanilla. Add flour mixture and mix well. Stir in raisins, nuts, and wheat germ, if using. Stir in oats.
- Roll dough into balls and place 3 inches apart on greased or parchment paper lined baking sheet. Flatten slightly. Bake 10-12 minutes or until almost no imprint remains when touched lightly with finger. Cool a few minutes on baking sheet. Remove to wire rack and cool completely.
- Note: The first time my son made these by himself (at about age 10 or 11), he accidentally put in 2 teaspoons of vanilla instead of the 1 teaspoon the original recipe called for. The cookies tasted so much richer that now I make the same "mistake" every time.

246.   Oatmeal Chocolate Chunk Cookies Recipe

Serving: 30 | Prep: | Cook: 30mins |Ready in:

Ingredients

- 1 1/2 teaspoon vanilla extract
- 3 cups (720 mL) quick-cooking or old-fashioned oats, uncooked
- 1 1/2 cups (360 mL) flour

- 1 teaspoon baking soda
- 1 teaspoon salt
- chocolate chunks, chips, or M&M-type candies to preference
- 1 cup (2 sticks - 300 mL) butter
- 3/4 cup (180 mL) brown sugar (original calls for light, but I only have dark available, and it works fine so long as you differentiate "done" and "burnt" from the colors)
- 1/2 cup (120 mL) granulated sugar
- 1 egg

Direction

- Preheat oven to 190C/375F.
- In large bowl cream butter and sugars until light and fluffy.
- Beat in egg and vanilla.
- In medium bowl combine oats, flour, baking soda and salt.
- Blend into creamed mixture.
- Stir in chocolate evenly.
- Drop by rounded tablespoon about 2 inches apart onto ungreased cookie sheets, or put in a casserole dish/bread pan to make cookie bars.
- Bake 8 to 9 minutes or until set.
- If making bars, give about 3-4 minutes to set before cutting them, then a few more minutes before transferring them to a plate or container.

247.   Oatmeal Cranberry White Chocolate Chunk Cookies Recipe

Serving: 30 | Prep: | Cook: 10mins |Ready in:

Ingredients

- 2/3 cup butter
- 2/3 cup light brown sugar
- 2 large eggs
- 1 1/2 cup old-fashioned rolled oats
- 1 1/2 cup flour

- 1 teasp. baking soda
- 1/2 teasp. salt
- 1 (6 oz.) package craisins.....the orginal flavor.. diced
- 2/3 cup white chocolate chunks or chips
- ....
- ****I would have to add some Pecans****

Direction

- Using an electric mixer beat butter and sugar in medium size bowl until light and fluffy
- Add eggs, mix well
- In separate bowl combine oats, flour, baking soda, and salt
- Add to butter mixture in several additions, mixing well after each
- Stir in dried cranberries and chocolate chunks
- Drop by rounded teaspoon unto an ungreased cookie sheet
- Bake at 375' F for 10-12 minutes or until golden brown
- Cool on wire rack.
- approx. 30 cookies

---

248.   Oatmeal Icebox Cookies Recipe

Serving: 36 | Prep: | Cook: 10mins | Ready in:

Ingredients

- 3/4 cup flour ; sifted
- 1/2 teaspoon salt
- 1/2 teaspoon baking soda
- 1/2 cup butter
- 1/2 cup firmly packed brown sugar
- 1/2 cup sugar
- 1 egg ; lightly beaten
- 1 teaspoon vanilla
- 1 1/2 cups quick-cooking oats
- 1/2 cup pecans ; finely chopped

Direction

- Sift together dry ingredients, set aside.
- Cream butter and sugars until fluffy.
- Beat in egg and vanilla; mix in dry ingredients, oats and nuts.
- Divide dough in half, turn out onto lightly floured board, and shape into 2 rolls about 10" long and 1 1/2" in diameter.
- Wrap in foil or plastic wrap and chill well or freeze.
- About 10 minutes before cookies are to be baked, preheat oven to 375 degrees.
- Slice rolls 1/4" thick and arrange cookies 2" apart on lightly greased baking sheet.
- Bake about 10 minutes, until tan.
- Cool 5 minutes on baking sheet, then transfer to wire rack to cool.
- Makes about 6 dozen cookies.
- NOTES: You can also use walnuts or toasted almonds instead of pecans.

---

249.   Oatmeal Kiss Cookies Recipe

Serving: 72 | Prep: | Cook: 10mins | Ready in:

Ingredients

- 1/2 cup butter, softened
- 1/2 cup shortening
- 1 cup sugar
- 1 cup packed brown sugar
- 2 eggs
- 2 cups all-purpose flour
- 1 teaspoon baking soda
- 1 teaspoon salt
- 2-1/4 cups quick-cooking oats
- 1 cup chopped nuts
- 72 milk chocolate kisses

Direction

- In a mixing bowl, cream the butter, shortening and sugars. Add eggs, one at a time, beating well after each addition.

- Combine the flour, baking soda and salt; gradually add to creamed mixture. Stir in oats and nuts. Roll into 1-in. balls. Place 2 in. apart on ungreased baking sheets.
- Bake at 375° for 10-12 minutes or until lightly browned. Immediately
- Press a chocolate kiss in the centre of each cookie. Remove to wire racks.

250. Oatmeal Lace Cookies Recipe

Serving: 8 | Prep: | Cook: 12mins | Ready in:

Ingredients

- 1 stick butter or 11/2 stick margerine
- 11/2 cups quick oats
- 1 tsp vanilla
- 1 tsp baking powder
- 3/4 cup sugar
- 1 tbsp flour
- 1 egg slightly beaten
- pinch of salt
- raisins (optional)

Direction

- Melt butter or margarine, pour over oats in a large bowl
- Mix sugar and flour
- Add all other ingredients to oat mixture
- Mix well
- Drop by spoonfuls onto the foiled baking sheet
- Bake @ 350 approx. 12 mins
- Let cool before removing from foil

251. Oatmeal Raisin Frost Bites Recipe

Serving: 4 | Prep: | Cook: 12mins | Ready in:

Ingredients

- 3/4 cup raisins
- 3 Tbs orange juice
- 1/2 cup butter at room temp
- 3/4 cup sugar
- 1 large egg
- 2 tsp orange peel-grated
- 1 cup all purpose flour
- 1 tsp baking soda
- 1 1/2 cup rolled oats
- 8 oz pkg white chocolate chips
- 1 tsp veg oil

Direction

- In a small bowl, combine orange juice and raisins; let stand overnight.
- In large bowl, beat butter and sugar until fluffy. Beat in egg and orange peel
- In another bowl, combine flour and baking soda
- Stir into butter mixture.
- Add raisins and nay soaking liquid and oats; mix well
- Drop dough by rounded teaspoonful onto greased baking sheets, spacing about 2 inches apart; flatten slightly.
- Bake at 350 for 10 to 12 minutes.
- Transfer to racks to cool completely
- In a small deep microwave-safe bowl, heat chocolate and oil 3-4 minutes on low power stirring once. Let stand 2 minutes. Stir until smooth. Dip one third of the cookie in chocolate. Set on waxed paper baking sheets. Chill until chocolate is firm.

252. Oatmeal Scotchies Recipe

Serving: 12 | Prep: | Cook: 7mins | Ready in:

Ingredients

- 1 1/4 cups all-purpose flour
- 1 teaspoon baking soda

- 1/2 teaspoon salt
- 1/2 teaspoon ground cinnamon
- 1 cup (2 sticks) butter or margarine
- 3/4 cup granulated sugar
- 3/4 cup packed brown sugar
- 2 large eggs
- 1 teaspoon vanilla extract or grated peel of 1 orange
- 3 cups quick or old-fashioned oats
- 1 2/3 cups (11-oz. pkg.) NESTLÉ® TOLL HOUSE® butterscotch Flavored Morsels

Direction

- PREHEAT oven to 375° F.
- COMBINE flour, baking soda, salt and cinnamon in small bowl.
- Beat butter, granulated sugar, brown sugar, eggs and vanilla extract in large mixer bowl.
- Gradually beat in flour mixture.
- Stir in oats and morsels.
- Drop by rounded tablespoon onto ungreased baking sheets.
- BAKE for 7 to 8 minutes for chewy cookies or 9 to 10 minutes for crisp cookies.
- Cool on baking sheets for 2 minutes; remove to wire racks to cool completely.
- PAN COOKIE VARIATION:
- Grease 15 x 10-inch jelly-roll pan.
- Prepare dough as above.
- Spread into prepared pan.
- Bake for 18 to 22 minutes or until light brown.
- Cool completely in pan on wire rack.
- Makes 4 dozen bars.

253. Oh Henry Bars Recipe

Serving: 18 | Prep: | Cook: 20mins | Ready in:

Ingredients

- 2/3 cup butter
- 1 cup brown sugar firmly packed
- 1 tablespoon vanilla
- 1/2 cup light corn syrup

- 4 cups quick oats
- 1 cup chocolate chips
- 2/3 cup chunky peanut butter

Direction

- Cream butter and sugar.
- Add vanilla, corn syrup and oats.
- Pat dough into lightly greased rectangular baking pan.
- Bake at 350 for 15 minutes.
- While dough is baking melt chocolate chips and peanut butter together over low heat.
- Cool dough slightly then spread chocolate mixture on top.
- Cool further then cut into bars.

254. Old Fashion Butter Cookies Recipe

Serving: 72 | Prep: | Cook: 5mins | Ready in:

Ingredients

- 1 cup butter
- 3/4 cup sugar
- 1 egg
- 2 TBSP. milk
- 1/2 teasp. vanilla
- 3 cups sifted flour
- 1 teasp. baking powder
- 1/2 teasp. salt

Direction

- Cream together using electric mixer set on cream setting (low) butter and sugar
- Stir in on cookie setting (medium) egg, milk, and vanilla
- Mix together the flour, baking powder and salt
- Add slowly to the butter mixture. Mix well
- Chill: 4 hours even better if you freeze the dough for a couple of days
- Divide dough into 1/3's first.

- Flour surface and roll out dough to 1/8 to 1/4 inch thick. Keep the other 2 doughs in the refrigerator
- Cut into circles. Place on an ungreased cookie sheet
- Bake at 375 to 400' F for 5 - 8 mins. or until very lightly brown

255. Old Fashioned Hedgehog Cake Recipe

Serving: 16 | Prep: | Cook: 1mins | Ready in:

Ingredients

- 4 oz butter
- 4 oz sugar
- 1 egg
- 1 tsp vanilla essence
- 1 Tbsp cocoa powder (heaped)
- 180g packet plain biscuits (like arrowroot, or milk coffee etc)
- 1 cup icing sugar
- pink food colouring

Direction

- Break up the biscuits into like...I dunno...half-centimeter sized chunks... (NOT crushed like you would for a cheesecake base).
- In a medium saucepan, cream together the butter and sugar, then mix in the egg and cocoa.
- Bring to boil for one minute (stirring). Remove from heat.
- Add the broken biscuits and mix it all up good.
- Transfer mixture to a lined slice tin, press it down firmly.
- Mix up your pink icing and spread it over the top.
- Put it in the fridge to cool... a few hours.
- Cut into like... fingers to serve.

256. Older Than The Hills Butter Cookies Recipe

Serving: 0 | Prep: | Cook: 1hours | Ready in:

Ingredients

- 2 cups salted butter, softened
- 2 cups powdered sugar
- 4 cups flour(slightly more or less, possibly)
- For butter Cream Frosting
- 1 stick salted butter, softened
- 3-4 cups powdered sugar
- 2t vanilla
- 4-6T half and half, cream or milk, depending on desired consistency
- baking goodies like sprinkles or candies(optional)

Direction

- For Butter Cookies
- Cream butter with sugar. Beat until light and fluffy.
- Add flour a little at a time until a stiff workable dough forms.
- Let refrigerate at about 15 minutes.
- Roll cookies out on a clean, dry surface with a little flour, if needed, to avoid sticking. Roll out to between 1/4-1/2 inch sheet.
- Cut with metal cookie cutters.
- Place on prepared baking sheet (parchment works best) or a baking stone (this is what I use)
- Bake in a preheated 350 oven for 12-14 minutes until edges are just starting to turn golden.
- Let cookies cool at least 15 minutes on the pan then carefully remove to a cooling rack to cool completely.
- Ice cookies when completely cooled.
- For Butter Cream Frosting
- Beat butter with vanilla and carefully add powdered sugar alternating with a T at a time of cream and mix well. Continue until desired

consistency is achieved. I don't do the smooth perfect iced cookies, because we like the more rustic look, it's what we remember but, you could ice these cookies with any favorite glaze or icing, if desired.

- Decorate as desired.
- **this cookie dough can also be rolled into a log, chilled well, and sliced to bake rather than rolling out to ice and decorate.

257. One Bowl White Chocolate Raspberry Chewy Bars Testing Recipe

Serving: 12 | Prep: | Cook: 35mins | Ready in:

Ingredients

- 3-4 (1 ounce) squares white chocolate or a heaping third-1/2 of a cup white chocolate chips
- 1 stick butter
- 1 2/3 cups white sugar
- 1 teaspoon vanilla
- 2 tsp baking powder
- 1/2 tsp salt
- 3 eggs
- 1 1/2 cups all-purpose flour
- 1 cup fresh or frozen red raspberries, about 6oz (if they are large it might be best to brake them into 3rds)
- optional-melted white chocolate to drizzle on top

Direction

- Preheat oven to 350 degrees F (180 degrees C).
- Microwave chocolate and butter in large bowl at HIGH for 1-2 minutes or until butter is melted.
- Stir until chocolate is melted.
- Add each ingredient, one at a time, in the order listed, and stirring (by hand) after each ingredient is added. Carefully fold in raspberries last.

- Spread in greased 13 x 9 inch pan. Bake for 35-40 minutes (do not over bake).
- After cooling at least 30 minutes. Melt optional chocolate and drizzle in crisscross pattern.

258. One Pot Cookie Mix Recipe

Serving: 25 | Prep: | Cook: 11mins | Ready in:

Ingredients

- 1 lb. butter or margarine
- 2 cups brown sugar
- 2 cups white sugar
- 2 cups oatmeal
- 2 cups wheaties
- 4 eggs
- 2 tsp. vanilla
- 4 1/3 cups flour
- 2 tsp. baking powder
- 2 tsp. soda
- 1 tsp salt
- 1 cup coconut
- l lg. pkg. chocolate chips
- 1/2 cup nuts

Direction

- In large bowl melt the butter or margarine.
- Add the remaining ingredients.
- Mix well.
- Drop about 1 TBS of cookie dough for each cookie on cookie sheet and bake at 350* for 10 to 12 min.

259. Orange Marmalade Cheese Bars Recipe

Serving: 12 | Prep: | Cook: 30mins | Ready in:

Ingredients

- 1 package orange cake mix
- 1/3 cup butter melted
- 1 egg
- 12 ounce jar orange marmalade
- 8 ounce package cream cheese softened
- 1/4 cup granulated sugar
- 1/2 teaspoon vanilla
- 1 egg

Direction

- Preheat oven to 350 then grease a rectangular pan.
- In a large bowl combine cake mix, butter and egg then mix with fork until just crumbly.
- Gently spoon 1-1/2 cups into measuring cup and set aside for topping.
- Press remainder of crumb mixture into bottom of pan and bake 10 minutes.
- Spread marmalade over baked crust.
- In a small bowl combine cream cheese, sugar, vanilla and egg then beat until smooth.
- Spread over preserves then sprinkle reserved topping mix over cream cheese mixture.
- Bake 30 minutes then chill and cut into squares.
- Store leftovers in refrigerator.

260.   Orange Slice Cookies Recipe

Serving: 24 | Prep: | Cook: 30mins | Ready in:

Ingredients

- 1 Pound orange slice candy
- 3/4 cup chopped nuts
- 2 and3/4 cup flour
- 4 eggs
- 2/3 cup butter
- 1 pound brown sugar

Direction

- Grease a12x18 in. pan

- Preheat oven to 325 degrees
- Cut candy into small pieces
- Dust candy and nuts with part of the flour
- Cream together the eggs, butter and brown sugar.
- Add flour mixture and mix until all flour is blended.
- Stir in candy and nuts until well mixed
- Spread in prepared pan and bake 30 minutes
- Cut into squares while hot.

261.   Oreo Cream Cheese Delights Recipe

Serving: 24 | Prep: | Cook: 5mins | Ready in:

Ingredients

- 1 bag Oreo cookies
- 8 ounce package cream cheese softened
- 12 ounces chocolate chips

Direction

- Crush cookies and combine with cream cheese.
- Shape into balls and refrigerate at least one hour.
- Melt chocolate chips then dip balls into melted chocolate.

262.   Oreo Something Or Others Recipe

Serving: 830 | Prep: | Cook: 5mins | Ready in:

Ingredients

- Package of Oreos or like cookie
- bananas
- peanut butter, any kind you prefer

- chocolate chips or chunks for melting. Again, any kind you prefer, dark, light white.

Direction

- Unscrew an Oreo. This doesn't have to be perfect, just don't break the Oreo. Sometimes using a paring knife is the best option.
- Put a pat of peanut butter in. I prefer crunchy.
- One slice of banana. I think the thicker the better, but it has to fit!
- Dip it in melted chocolate and let set.
- Go back and drizzle a different kind of chocolate across them to make them prettier if you prefer.

---

263.   Outrageous Rocky Road Squares Recipe

Serving: 12 | Prep: | Cook: |Ready in:

Ingredients

- 2 cups chocolate chips (I use the equivalent in really good quality chocolate)
- 1 can sweetened condensed milk
- 2 Tbsp butter
- 2 cups peanuts
- 1 package mini marshmallows

Direction

- Heat first three ingredients in a bowl in the microwave, stirring frequently until smooth and melted.
- Let cool slightly
- Add peanuts and marshmallows
- Press into parchment paper lined 9 x 13 inch pan and let cool in the fridge until cold.
- Cut into squares.
- Freezes well.

---

264.   PEANUT BUTTER CRISPS Recipe

Serving: 28 | Prep: | Cook: 12mins |Ready in:

Ingredients

- 1 C. butter or margarine, softened
- 1/2 C.creamy peanut butter
- 1/2 C. sugar
- 1/2 C. firmly packed brown sugar
- 1 egg
- 1 tsp. vanilla extract
- 1 1/3 C. all-purpose flour
- 3 1/2 C. corn flakes, finely crushed, or 1 cup corn flake crumbs
- salted peanuts

Direction

- Combine butter and peanut butter in a large mixing bowl, creaming well.
- Add sugar, and beat well; add egg and vanilla, mixing well.
- Gradually add flour, and beat well.
- Cover dough tightly, and refrigerate several hours or overnight.
- Shape dough into 1 inch balls; roll each in corn flake crumbs.
- Press one peanut in centre of each.
- Place on a greased cookie sheet; bake at 350° for 12 minutes or until cookies are lightly browned.
- Yield: about 5 dozen.

---

265.   PEANUT BUTTER KISS COOKIES Recipe

Serving: 12 | Prep: | Cook: 10mins |Ready in:

Ingredients

- peanut butter KISS cookies
- 1 c. peanut butter
- 1 c. sugar

- 1 egg
- 1 t. vanilla
- 24 milk chocolate kisses

Direction

- In a mixing bowl, cream peanut butter and sugar. Add the egg and vanilla; beat until well blended.
- Roll into 1 1/4 inch balls.
- Place 2 inches apart on ungreased cookie sheet.
- Bake at 350degrees for 10-12 minutes or until tops are slightly cracked.
- Immediately press one chocolate kiss into the centre of each cookie. Cool for 5 minutes before removing from pans to wire rack. Yields 2 dozen.
- *** If you want a plain cookie, just roll them in balls then roll the balls in sugar, crisscross with a fork and bake. Good either way.

266.   PEANUT BUTTER SQUARES Recipe

Serving: 6 | Prep: | Cook: |Ready in:

Ingredients

- 1 cup peanut butter
- 1 cup icing sugar
- 1 1/2 cups Rice Krispies
- 3 tbsp soft margerine
- chocolate ice cream topping for drizzle
- 2 tbsp flaked coconut

Direction

- Mix all ingredients together except drizzle & coconut.
- Pat down in an 8x8 pan.
- Drizzle chocolate on and sprinkle with coconut
- Cut & serve

267.   PEPPERMINT SNOWBALL COOKIES Recipe

Serving: 36 | Prep: | Cook: 12mins |Ready in:

Ingredients

- Candy Coating:
- 1/4 c. Finely crushed peppermint candies
- 1/4 c. Confectioner's' sugar
- cookie Dough:
- 1/4 c. Finely crushed peppermint candies
- 1/3 c. Confectioner's' sugar
- 1 c. butter, softened
- 1 tsp. vanilla
- 2 1/4 c. flour
- 1/4 tsp. salt

Direction

- Preheat oven to 325* Mix 1/4 c. Crushed candies and 1/4 c. Confectioner's' sugar, set aside.
- In separate bowl, mix butter, 1/3 c. Confectioner's' sugar, 1/4 c. Crushed candies and vanilla. Stir in flour and salt. Shape dough by scooping into teaspoonful-sized balls. Place 2" apart on an ungreased cookie sheet. Bake 12-15 minutes. Immediately remove from cookie sheet and roll in candy mixture. Cool and eat.

268.   PINEAPPLE CHEESECAKE SQUARES Recipe

Serving: 10 | Prep: | Cook: 10mins |Ready in:

Ingredients

- Pat in pan crust
- 2 packages cream cheese (8 oz each)
- 1/2 cup sugar

- eggs
- 2/3 cup unsweetened pineapple juice
- 1/4 cup flour
- 1/4 cup sugar
- 1 cup Crsh pineapple(20 oz)drained
- 1 cup juice from drained can(save)
- 1/2 cup whipping cream

Direction

- Heat oven to 350deg. Bake crust. Beat cream cheese in bowl until smooth and fluffy; beat in 1/2 cup sugar and the eggs. Stir in 2/3 cup juice. Pour cream cheese mixture over hot crust. Bake just until centre is set, about 20 minutes. Cool completely. Mix flour and 1/4 cup sugar in 2 qt. saucepan. Stir in 1 cup of saved Pineapple juice. Heat to boiling over medium heat, stirring constantly. Boil and stir 1 minute. Remove from heat; fold in drained pineapple. Cool completely. Beat whipping cream in chilled bowl until stiff. Fold into pineapple mixture. Spread carefully over dessert. Cover loosely and refrigerate until firm, about 4 hours. Cut into squares.

269. Party Bars Recipe

Serving: 48 | Prep: | Cook: 35mins | Ready in:

Ingredients

- BOTTOM LAYER
- 2 cups flour
- 2 tsp. baking soda
- 2 cups brown sugar, packed
- 1/2 cup margarine
- 1 cup coconut
- 1 cup oats
- TOP LAYER
- 4 eggs
- 2 cups chocolate chips
- 1 cup brown sugar, packed
- 1 cup chopped walnuts
- 1/2 cup margarine

- 2 tbls. flour

Direction

- Sift flour and baking soda.
- Mix brown sugar and margarine until crumbly.
- Stir into flour, add coconut and oats.
- Press firmly into a 9x13 pan.
- Mix eggs, chocolate chips, brown sugar, walnuts, margarine and flour.
- Pour over base.
- Bake at 350 degrees for 35 minutes.

270. Pastry Squares Recipe

Serving: 24 | Prep: | Cook: 30mins | Ready in:

Ingredients

- 4 cups flour
- 2 T sugar
- 2 sticks oleomargarine (shortening) equals 1 cup, at room temp
- 1 pkg yeast
- 1/4 cup warm water
- 2/3 cup warm milk
- 2 cans pie filling - same or 2 different kinds

Direction

- Do not use mixer. Blend flour, sugar and oleo with pastry blender. Blend well. Dissolve yeast in water and add milk. Add to flour mixture and mix well. Divide dough into 2 pieces - one a bit larger than the other. Roll out the smaller one to size of pan. Place in ungreased 15" x 10" pan and pat to shape and up sides. Let rest for 15 minutes. Spread on pie filling - one can at each end of pan. Roll out the larger one, while the other dough is resting, to size of pan also - don't have to be real particular. Place over top - does not have to be sealed. Bake at 350 degrees for 30 minutes. When cooled frost or glaze. Cut. Rough edges can be trimmed off.

271.   Paula Deens Red Velvet Sandwich Cookies Recipe

Serving: 6 | Prep: | Cook: 10mins |Ready in:

Ingredients

- 1 1/3 cups all-purpose flour
- 2 tablespoons cocoa powder
- 1 teaspoon baking powder
- 1/4 teaspoon baking soda
- 1/2 teaspoon salt
- 1/4 cup butter, room temperature
- 1 cup sugar
- 2 eggs
- 2 tablespoons buttermilk
- 2 teaspoons apple cider vinegar
- 1 teaspoon vanilla extract
- 1 tablespoon red food coloring
- For the Cream Cheese Frosting:
- 1 pound cream cheese, softened
- 2 sticks butter, softened
- 1 teaspoon vanilla extract
- 4 cups powdered sugar
- 3/4 cup finely chopped pecans, optional

Direction

- Preheat oven to 375 degrees F.
- Mix together flour, cocoa powder, baking powder, baking soda and salt in a small bowl.
- Cream together the butter and sugar until light and fluffy, about 3 minutes.
- Add the eggs 1 at a time.
- Then beat in the buttermilk, vinegar, vanilla and red food coloring. Once combined, add the dry ingredients to wet.
- Mix until thoroughly combined.
- Onto a parchment lined sheet tray, drop batter using an ice cream scoop, forming 2-inch round circles.
- Bake for 10 minutes, until baked through.
- Cookies should be cake-like and light.

- Allow to cool for a few minutes on the baking sheet, then remove to a wire rack to cool completely.
- For the Cream Cheese Frosting:
- In a large mixing bowl, beat the cream cheese, butter, and vanilla together until smooth.
- Add the sugar and on low speed, beat until incorporated.
- Increase the speed to high and mix until very light and fluffy.
- Spread the cream cheese frosting between 2 cooled cookies and roll the edges in finely chopped pecans, if desired.

272.   Paw Cookies Recipe

Serving: 30 | Prep: | Cook: 30mins |Ready in:

Ingredients

- 1 cup (2 sticks) butter or margarine, softened
- 1-1/2 cups firmly packed brown sugar
- 2 eggs
- 1 tsp vanilla
- 2 cups flour
- 1 tsp baking soda
- 4 cups POST GOLDEN CRISP cereal, divided
- 8 squares BAKER'S Semi-Sweet baking chocolate

Direction

- PREHEAT oven to 350°F.
- Beat butter and sugar in large bowl with electric mixer on medium speed until light and fluffy.
- Blend in eggs and vanilla.
- Add flour and baking soda; mix well.
- Stir in 3 cups of the cereal.
- DROP heaping teaspoonful of dough, 2 inches apart, onto ungreased baking sheets.
- BAKE 8 to 10 min. or until golden brown.
- Remove from baking sheets to wire racks; cool completely.

- Dip cooled cookies halfway into melted chocolate; immediately sprinkle with remaining 1 cup cereal to resemble bear paws.
- Place on wax paper-lined tray.
- Let stand until chocolate is firm.
- Store in tightly covered container at room temperature.
- Makes about 5 dozen cookies

273. Peach Streusel Bars Recipe

Serving: 16 | Prep: | Cook: 40mins | Ready in:

Ingredients

- 2 cups all-purpose flour
- 1/2 cup firmly packed light brown sugar
- 1 teaspoon grated lemon rind
- 1/4 teaspoon ground nutmeg
- 1/4 teaspoon salt
- 3/4 cup (1 1/2 sticks) unsalted butter
- 1 12-ounce jar peach preserves

Direction

- Preheat oven to 375 degrees.
- Grease 9- by 9- by 2-inch square pan.
- Combine flour, sugar, lemon rind, nutmeg and salt in large bowl. Cut in butter with pastry blender until mixture is crumbly. Reserve 1 cup. Pat remaining mixture evenly into prepared pan.
- Spread preserves evenly over dough, leaving 1/4-inch border around edge. Sprinkle with reserved flour mixture.
- Bake for 40 minutes or until lightly browned. Cool in PAN on wire rack.
- Cut into bite-sized bars. Store for up to 1 week in air-tight container.
- I refrigerate mine so they don't mold and take them out to warm up before eating.
- Makes 16 bars.
- 2001 Countdown to Christmas-St Pete Times

274. Peanut Butter And Jelly Cookies Recipe

Serving: 25 | Prep: | Cook: 12mins | Ready in:

Ingredients

- 4 tablespoons unsalted butter, soft
- ½ cup white sugar
- ½ cup brown sugar
- 1 cup peanut butter, creamy or chunky (I use Adams brand)
- 1 each whole egg
- 1 ¼ cup unbleached all purpose flour
- ¼ teaspoon kosher salt
- 1 tablespoon baking powder
- jam or jelly, according to your preference

Direction

- Cream together butter and sugars until mixture is light and fluffy.
- Beat in peanut butter until uniformly combined.
- Beat in egg.
- Stir in dry ingredients and mix until dough comes together. Dough will likely be a bit crumbly at the bottom of the bowl; just knead a few times to mix it in. Wrap dough in plastic and chill at least thirty minutes. Preheat oven to 350°F.
- Divide dough into ½ ounce pieces and roll into spheres.
- Place balls on baking sheet (greased, or lined with parchment or a Silpat) and smash to form discs about ¼" tall.
- Using your finger, a chopstick, or some other similarly shaped item, press a divot in the dough large enough to accommodate ⅛- ¼ teaspoon jam or jelly.
- Spoon preserves into the dough (I use a heaped ⅛ teaspoon).
- Sprinkle white sugar around the edge of the cookie, if you'd like a crispier finish.

- Bake in preheated oven for 8 - 12 minutes, or until edges are firm and golden.

275. Peanut Butter Balls In Chocolate Recipe

Serving: 20 | Prep: | Cook: | Ready in:

Ingredients

- 2 Cups peanut butter
- 1 cup butter
- 5 cups powdered sugar
- 1 tsp. vanilla
- 1 or 2 squares of Baker's sweet chocolate

Direction

- Mix butters and vanilla together.
- Slowly mix in powdered sugar.
- Form into balls.
- Melt 1 or 2 squares of Baker's sweet chocolate (or your favorite sweet chocolate).
- Dip balls in chocolate and chill.

276. Peanut Butter Bars 1 Recipe

Serving: 12 | Prep: | Cook: | Ready in:

Ingredients

- 4 Cups - creamy peanut butter
- 1/2 Cup - Softened butter (margerine if 80% vegetable oil)
- 2 Teaspoons - vanilla
- 4 Cups - powdered sugar (sifting recommended)
- 1/3 Cup - brown sugar, packed
- 1 1/2 - 2 Cups (9 - 12 ounces) - milk chocolate Pieces

Direction

- In a large mixing bowl beat Peanut Butter, Butter, and Vanilla with an electric mixer.
- Gradually blend in Confectioners' Sugar and Brown Sugar until combined (occasionally scraping sides of bowl).
- Spread in a 13 x 9 x 2 inch pan and set aside (lining with foil or wax paper will make removal easier).
- Melt Milk Chocolate Pieces in a microwave-safe bowl on medium for 3 - 4 minutes or until melted (stirring once or twice).
- Spread melted chocolate evenly over peanut butter mixture.
- Cover and chill for 2 hours or overnight. ENJOY!!!
- (Serves 12 - 24)

277. Peanut Butter Bars Recipe

Serving: 2 | Prep: | Cook: 30mins | Ready in:

Ingredients

- 1/2 c peanut butter
- 1 stick of margarine
- 1 1/2 cu sugar
- 2 eggs
- 1t vanilla
- 1 c lily white self rising flour

Direction

- Preheat oven to 350 degrees
- Grease and flour 13x9x2 inch pan
- Melt peanut butter and margarine in butter for 1 minute
- Add remaining ingredients and stir till well blended
- Bake for 25-30 minutes
- Let cool then cut into bars

278. Peanut Butter Bars With Chips Recipe

Serving: 32 | Prep: | Cook: 30mins | Ready in:

Ingredients

- 1 pkg (19.5) package of a good brownie mix (plain not with nuts)
- 2 eggs
- 1/3 cup cooking oil
- 1 cup chopped peanuts
- 1 (14 oz) sweetened condensed milk
- 1/2 cup peanut butter (smooth)
- 1/2 (12 oz) pkg of peanut butter/chocolate swirl chips

Direction

- Preheat oven to 350
- Lightly grease a 9 x 13 baking dish, set aside
- In large bowl combine brownie mix, eggs and oil.
- Beat with electric mixer on medium speed until combined
- Stir in peanuts
- Pour half the batter into prepared pan, spreading evenly
- In another bowl, whisk together peanut butter and condensed milk
- Spread evenly of brownie mixture in pan
- Top with half of the chips
- Put the saved brownie mixture in clumps over chips and with fingers
- Spread out in pan
- Top with remaining chips
- Bake in oven 25-30 minutes or until top is set and edges lightly browned
- Remove, cool in pan on wire rack.
- When completely cool, but into bars
- Storing: layer bars between wax paper in airtight container

279. Peanut Butter Buckeye Bars Recipe

Serving: 1 | Prep: | Cook: 30mins | Ready in:

Ingredients

- 1 (18.25 or 18.5 oz) package chocolate cake mix
- 1/4 cup vegetable oil
- 1 egg
- 1 cup chopped peanuts
- 1 (14oz) can sweetened condensed milk (NOT evaporated)
- 1/2 cup peanut butter (Favorite!!)

Direction

- Preheat oven to 350 degrees F (325 degrees for a glass dish)
- In large bowl, combine cake mix, oil and egg; beat on medium speed until crumbly. Stir in peanuts.
- Reserving 1 1/2 cups crumb mixture, press remainder on bottom of greased 13x9 inch baking pan.
- In medium bowl, beat sweetened condensed milk and peanut butter until smooth; spread over prepared crust.
- Sprinkle with reserved crumb mixture.
- Bake 25 - 30 minutes or until set.
- Cool and cut into bars.
- Store loosely covered at room temperature.
- **
- -It try to avoid looking forward or backward; and try to keep looking upward- Charlotte Bronte
- **

280. Peanut Butter Caramel Bars Recipe

Serving: 1 | Prep: | Cook: 25mins | Ready in:

Ingredients

- 1 pkg. (18 oz) yellow cake mix
- 1/2 C. butter softened
- 1 egg
- 20 miniature peanut butter cups chopped
- 2 T. cornstarch
- 1 (12 1/4 oz) jar caramel ice cream topping
- 1/4 C. peanut butter
- 1/2 C. salted peanuts
- Topping:
- 1 (16 oz) can milk chocolate frosting
- 1/2 C. chopped salted peanuts

Direction

- In a mixing bowl, combine the dry cake mix, butter and egg; beat until no longer crumbly, about 3 minutes.
- Stir in the peanut butter cups.
- Press into a greased 9x13 baking pan.
- Bake at 350 for 18-22 minutes or until lightly browned.
- Meanwhile, in a saucepan, combine cornstarch, caramel topping and peanut butter until smooth. Cook over low heat, stirring occasionally until mixture comes to a boil, about 25 minutes. Cook and stir 1-2 minutes longer.
- Remove from the heat; stir in peanuts. Spread evenly over warm crust. Bake 6-7 minutes longer or until almost set.
- Cool completely on a wire rack.
- Spread with frosting; sprinkle with peanuts.
- Refrigerate for at least 1 hour before cutting. Store in refrigerator.

281. Peanut Butter Clouds Recipe

Serving: 1 | Prep: | Cook: 12mins | Ready in:

Ingredients

- 1 cup shortening
- 1 cup peanut butter
- 1 cup granulated sugar
- 1 cup confectioner's sugar
- 2 eggs
- 1 teaspoon vanilla
- 2 cups all-purpose flour -- sifted
- 3 teaspoons baking soda
- 1 teaspoon salt

Direction

- Preheat oven to 350 F.
- Cream the shortening, peanut butter, and sugars together. Beat in eggs and vanilla.
- Sift the flour, soda and salt together, and add gradually to the creamed mixture. Beat well.
- Drop from a teaspoon onto ungreased cookie sheets. Flatten with a floured fork.
- Bake at 350 F. for 12 to 15 minutes.

282. Peanut Butter Cookies Recipe

Serving: 24 | Prep: | Cook: 40mins | Ready in:

Ingredients

- 1 1/2 cups all-purpose flour
- 1 teaspoon baking soda
- 1/2 teaspoon salt
- 1 cup creamy or chunky peanut butter
- 1/2 cup shortening
- 1 cup granulated sugar
- 1 large egg
- 1 teaspoon vanilla extract

Direction

- Preheat oven to 400 degrees
- In a medium bowl sift to combine flour, baking soda and salt
- In a large bowl beat together peanut butter, shortening, and granulated sugar until smooth.
- Add in egg and vanilla
- Combine flour mixture with peanut butter mixture, scrapping the sides of the bowl to insure batter is well blended.
- Cover bowl with plastic and place in frig for 20 minutes
- Using a teaspoon drop batter 1 inch apart on an ungreased cookie sheet.
- Using a fork make crisscross pattern flattening cookies slightly.
- Bake for 10 to 12 minutes per your oven

283.   Peanut Butter Cookies With A Hint Of Orange Recipe

Serving: 10 | Prep: | Cook: 15mins | Ready in:

Ingredients

- 100g SR flour
- 50g castor sugar
- 50g butter or marg
- 3tbsp peanut butter
- 1 egg, beaten
- grated rind of half an orange
- 3tbsp brown sugar

Direction

- Preheat the oven to 180c
- Grease 2 baking trays
- Cream butter, orange rind, peanut butter, margarine and both sugars together until light and fluffy.
- Work in egg and stir in flour to form a firm mixture.
- Roll into walnut sized balls and space well apart on baking trays.
- Flatten with a large spatula until thin.

- Bake for 15mins until golden brown.

284.   Peanut Butter Crispy Bars Recipe

Serving: 9 | Prep: | Cook: 5mins | Ready in:

Ingredients

- peanut butter Crispy Bars
- For the crispy crust:
- 1 ¾ cups crisped rice cereal
- ¼ cup sugar
- 3 tablespoons light corn syrup
- 3 tablespoons unsalted butter, melted
- For the milk chocolate peanut butter layer:
- 5 ounces good-quality milk chocolate, coarsely chopped
- 1 cup creamy peanut butter
- For the chocolate icing:
- 3 ounces dark chocolate (60% to 72% cacao), coarsely chopped
- ½ teaspoon light corn syrup
- 4 tablespoons (1/2 stick) unsalted butter

Direction

- Make the crispy crust:
- Lightly spray a paper towel with non-stick spray and use it to rub the bottom and sides of an 8-inch square baking pan
- Put the cereal in a large bowl and set aside.
- Pour ¼ cup water into a small saucepan. Gently add the sugar and corn syrup (do not let any sugar or syrup get on the sides of the pan) and use a small wooden spoon to stir the mixture until just combined. Put a candy thermometer in the saucepan. Cook over medium-high heat and bring to a boil; cook until mixture reaches the soft ball stage, 235 degrees F.
- Remove from the heat, stir in the butter, and pour the mixture over the cereal. Working quickly, stir until the cereal is thoroughly coated, then pour it into the prepared pan.

Using your hands, press the mixture into the bottom of the pan (do not press up the sides. Let the crust cool to room temperature while you make the next layer.

- Make the milk chocolate peanut butter layer:
- In a large nonreactive metal bowl, stir together the chocolate and the peanut butter.
- Set the bowl over a saucepan of simmering water and cook, stirring with a rubber spatula, until the mixture is smooth. Remove the bowl from the pan and stir for about 30 seconds to cool slightly. Pour the mixture over the cooled crust. Put the pan in the refrigerator for 1 hour, or until the top layer hardens.
- Make the chocolate icing:
- In a large nonreactive metal bowl, combine the chocolate, corn syrup, and butter.
- Set the bowl over a saucepan of simmering water and cook, stirring with a rubber spatula, until the mixture is completely smooth. Remove the bowl from the pan and stir for 30 seconds to cool slightly. Pour the mixture over the chilled milk chocolate peanut butter layer and spread into and even layer. Put the pan in the refrigerator for 1 hour or until the topping hardens.
- Cut into 9 squares and serve. The bars can be stored in the refrigerator, covered tightly, for up to 4 days.

---

285.   Peanut Butter And Jelly Bars Recipe

Serving: 24 | Prep: | Cook: 45mins |Ready in:

Ingredients

- 1 stick unsalted butter
- 1/2 cup sugar
- 1 large egg (room tempature
- 1/2 tsp vanilla extract
- 1 cup creamy peanut butter
- 1 1/2 cup all-purpose flour
- 1/2 tsp baking powder

- 1/2 tsp salt
- 1 1/2 cup strawberry preserves
- 2/3 cup salted peanuts
- 2/3 cup peanut butter chips

Direction

- Preheat oven to 350 degrees F. Butter and lightly flower a 9 x 13 baking pan.
- Using an electric mixer on medium speed, cream butter and sugar until light and fluffy. Lower speed and add egg, vanilla, and peanut butter. Beat.
- In a separate bowl sift flower, baking powder, and salt. On low speed, slowly add flour mixture to peanut butter mixture. Mix to make dough. Set aside 1/2 cup of dough.
- Using your fingertips, press remaining dough into an even layer in the pan. Spread preserves over dough. Crumble preserved 1/2 cup dough over preserves. Sprinkle with peanuts and peanut butter chips.
- Bake 45 minutes until golden and bubbly.
- Cool on wire rack and cut into bars.

---

286.   Peanut Cake Bars Recipe

Serving: 72 | Prep: | Cook: 13mins |Ready in:

Ingredients

- 1 (18 1/4 ounce) box chocolate cake mix
- 1/2 cup water
- 1/3 cup butter or margarine, softened
- 1 egg
- Topping
- 3 cups miniature marshmallows
- 1 (10 ounce) package peanut butter chips
- 2/3 cup light corn syrup
- 1/4 cup butter or margarine
- 2 teaspoons vanilla extract
- 2 cups crisp rice cereal
- 2 cups salted peanuts

Direction

- In a bowl, combine dry cake mix, water, butter and egg until blended.
- Press into a greased 15 x 10-inch baking pan. Bake at 350 degrees F for 13 to 16 minutes or until a wooden pick inserted near the center comes out clean. Sprinkle with marshmallows. Bake 2 minutes longer.
- Cool.
- TOPPING
- In a saucepan, combine peanut butter chips, corn syrup, butter and vanilla extract. Cook over low heat until melted; stir until smooth.
- Remove from the heat; stir in cereal and peanuts. Spoon over marshmallows.
- Cool before cutting.

287. Peanut Cheerios Bar Recipe

Serving: 6 | Prep: | Cook: 20mins | Ready in:

Ingredients

- 1/4 cup sugar
- 1/4 cup honey
- 1/4 cup peanut butter
- 1 1/2 cups cheerios
- 1/4 cup salted peanuts

Direction

- In a medium saucepan, combine the sugar and honey, Cook and stir over medium heat until sugar is dissolved. Remove from the heat, stir in peanut butter until blended. Add cheerios and peanuts. Stir to coat. Spread into an 8x4 loaf pan, coated with cooking spray. Cover and chill 1 hour before cutting...Makes 6 bars

288. Peanutty Buttery Squares Recipe

Serving: 24 | Prep: | Cook: 30mins | Ready in:

Ingredients

- 1 cup Karo® Light or with Real brown sugar corn syrup
- 1/2 cup (1 stick) butter
- 1 cup sugar
- 2-1/2 cups creamy peanut butter or 1 (18 ounce) jar peanut butter
- Mazola Pure™ canola oil cooking spray
- 7 ounces (about 7 cups) Kellogg's® Rice Krispies or your favorite ready-to-eat cereal
- Note: fruit Loops work well too but my favorite is Kellogg's® Rice Krispies.
- 1 cup chocolate chips
- 1 cup butterscotch chips

Direction

- In a large saucepan, combine Karo® syrup, sugar and butter over medium heat and bring to a boil.
- Reduce heat to simmer and stir in peanut butter until smooth.
- Remove pan from heat.
- Mix cereal thoroughly into peanut butter and pour into 13 x 9" pan sprayed with cooking spray.
- Refrigerate pan for 20 minutes.
- Melt chocolate chips and butterscotch chips over low heat and spread over the hardened peanut butter and cereal mixture.
- Place pan back in refrigerator for until hard.
- Chill Time: 30 minutes
- Makes 24 squares

289. Peanutty Candy Bars Recipe

Serving: 0 | Prep: | Cook: 15mins | Ready in:

Ingredients

- 4 cups quick-cooking oats
- 1 cup packed brown sugar
- 2/3 cup butter, melted
- 1/2 cup plus 2/3 cup peanut butter, divided
- 1/2 cup light corn syrup
- 1 tsp vanilla
- 1 pkg. (11 oz.) butterscotch chips
- 1 cup (6 oz.) semisweet chocolate chips
- 1 cup chopped salted peanuts

Direction

- In a large bowl, combine the oats, brown sugar, butter, 1/2 cup peanut butter, corn syrup, and the vanilla.
- Press into a greased 13 x 9 inch baking pan.
- Bake at 375 F for 12-14 minutes or until the mixture is bubbly around the edges.
- In a microwave-safe bowl, melt the butterscotch chips and the chocolate chips.
- Stir until smooth.
- Stir in the peanuts and the remaining peanut butter
- Spread over the oat mixture.
- Cool for 10 minutes
- Chill until set.

---

290.   Pecan Rocks Recipe

Serving: 48 | Prep: | Cook: 20mins | Ready in:

Ingredients

- 1/2 pound butter
- 1 cup sifted powdered sugar
- 1 teaspoon vanilla
- ½ pound (2 cups) chopped pecans
- 2 1/4 cups sifted flour

Direction

- Preheat oven to 350°.
- Cream butter thoroughly.

- Add powdered sugar, a little at a time.
- Beat until very light and fluffy.
- Add vanilla.
- Using a wooden spoon, add flour alternately with chopped nuts.
- Place mounds of dough onto a cookie sheet. Do not compress the dough. Just pat it gently to hold shape.
- Bake until golden brown, about 20 minutes. Watch carefully.
- Remove from baking sheet and cool on a wire rack.
- When cooled, dip cookies into powdered sugar.
- NOTE: You do not want to beat the flour into the butter. Incorporating the flour and nuts by hand is imperative. You also want to handle the dough as little as possible when forming the cookies. The dough may seem dry and seem as if the cookies won't hold shape, but they do.

---

291.   Pecan Butterscotch Cookies Recipe

Serving: 112 | Prep: | Cook: 9mins | Ready in:

Ingredients

- 1 cup compelete buttermilk biscuit mix
- 1 pkg.{3.4 oz.} instand butterscotch pudding mix{May use sugar free
- 1/3 cup butter melted
- 1 egg
- 1/2 cup chopped pecans toasted

Direction

- In a large bowl beat the biscuit mix pudding mix butter and egg till blended
- Stir in pecans
- Drop by tablespoonsful 2 inches apart onto greased baking sheet flatten with bottom of glass.

- Bake at 350 degrees 8-10 minutes until edges begin to brown remove to wire rack to cool

292. Pineapple Cookies Recipe

Serving: 48 | Prep: | Cook: 20mins | Ready in:

Ingredients

- 1/2 cup shortening
- 1/2 cup brown sugar
- 1/2 white sugar
- 1 egg, beaten
- 1/2 tsp. vanilla
- 2 cups flour
- 2 tsps. baking powder
- 1/4 tsp. baking soda
- 1/4 tsp. salt
- 1 cup crushed pineapple
- 2/3 cup chopped walnuts (optional)

Direction

- Cream shortening and sugars.
- Add beaten egg and vanilla.
- Add dry ingredients.
- Drain pineapple and add to mixture, then nuts and flavoring.
- Drop from teaspoon onto a greased baking sheet.
- Bake at 350 degrees for 15-20 minutes,
- Makes approximately 4 dozen

293. Pineapple Drop Cookies Recipe

Serving: 16 | Prep: | Cook: 15mins | Ready in:

Ingredients

- 2/3 cup shortening

- 1-1/4 cup granulated sugar
- 1 teaspoon vanilla extract
- 1/2 teaspoon pineapple extract
- 1 egg
- 2 cups all-purpose flour
- 2 teaspoons baking powder
- 1/4 teaspoon salt
- 3/4 cup crushed pineapple well drained
- 1/2 cup pecans chopped

Direction

- Cream shortening, sugar and flavorings then add egg and beat until smooth.
- Sift flour, baking powder and salt together.
- Add to egg mixture alternately with drained pineapple.
- Fold in pecans and drop by teaspoons 3" apart on ungreased cookie sheet.
- Bake at 350 for 15 minutes.

294. Pineapple Squares Recipe

Serving: 20 | Prep: | Cook: 50mins | Ready in:

Ingredients

- 3 small tins crushed pineapple
- 1 cup sugar
- 9 tbsp minute tapioca
- 1 lb Crisco
- 5 cups flour
- 1 tsp salt
- 1 cup milk
- icing
- 1/4 lb Philly cream cheese
- 1 lb icing sugar
- 2 tbsp milk
- and chopped walnuts to sprinkle on top

Direction

- You will need a large cookie sheet with deep sides to bake this in.
- Mix pineapple, sugar and tapioca and set aside

- Mix Crisco, flour, salt and milk to make pastry, then divide in 2
- Line bottom of pan with half, fill with pineapple mixture, and cover with other half
- Make sure to cut slits on top for steam to come out while baking
- Bake at 350 for 45-50 mins
- While still slightly warm put icing on and sprinkle with walnuts

295. Polish Cookies Galicyjskie Cookies Recipe

Serving: 24 | Prep: | Cook: 30mins | Ready in:

Ingredients

- 4 eggs, separated
- 1/2 cup cream
- 3-1/2 to 4 Tablespoons confectioners' sugar
- 1/2 to 1 teaspoon ground cinnamon
- 2-3/4 pounds potatoes - peeled, finely grated, and squeezed completely of any liquid
- 2 Tablespoons raisins, soaked in boiling water to plump (optional)
- 1 cup All Purpose flour
- 1 pinch salt
- 1 cup oil for deep frying
- Either plain confectioners' sugar for dusting or a mixture of cinnamon and confectioners' sugar.

Direction

- Beat together the egg yolks, cream 3 tablespoons confectioners' sugar, and cinnamon until smooth.
- Stir into the grated potatoes along with the raisins, and mix until well combined; then stir in the flour.
- Beat the egg whites with salt until stiff.
- Gently fold into the potato mixture.
- Heat oil to 350 degrees F (175 degrees C) in a deep fryer or electric skillet.

- Fry the dough by dropping heaping tablespoon-sized dollops into the hot oil.
- Fry until golden brown on both sides, then drain on paper towel.
- Dust with confectioners' sugar.
- Makes 24 cookies.

296. Potato Chip Cookies Recipe

Serving: 24 | Prep: | Cook: 12mins | Ready in:

Ingredients

- 1/2 cup of butter (softened)
- 1/2 cup sugar
- 3/4 cup flour
- 3/4 cup crushed potato chips
- 1 tsp. vanilla

Direction

- Cream butter and sugar add vanilla
- Add flour and chips.
- Mix well.
- Drop onto cookie sheet in small amounts.
- Bake at 350 degrees for 12 min.

297. Pumpkin Bars Recipe

Serving: 9 | Prep: | Cook: 30mins | Ready in:

Ingredients

- ¾ C flour
- ¾ tsp salt
- ½ tsp soda
- ½ tsp nutmeg
- ½ tsp cinnamon
- 2 eggs
- 1 C brown sugar
- 2/3 C canned pure pumpkin, not pie filling

- ¼ c oil
- ½ c nuts

Direction

- Beat eggs and sugar together, add oil: add sifted dry ingredients. Stir in pumpkin and nuts.
- Pour into 9 in square greased pan. Bake at 350 for about 30 mins. Cool 5 mins.
- Frost with cream cheese icing, your own or from a can.

298.   Pumpkin Cookies Recipe

Serving: 0 | Prep: | Cook: 10mins | Ready in:

Ingredients

- 1 cup sugar
- 1 cup canned pumpkin
- 1/2 cup shortening
- 2 cups flour
- 1 tsp. baking powder
- 1 tsp. baking soda
- 1/4 tsp salt
- 1 tsp. ground cinnamon
- 1/2 cup semi-sweet chocolate chips

Direction

- Heat oven to 375
- Mix sugar, pumpkin and shortening. Stir in flour, baking powder, baking soda, cinnamon, and salt. Stir in chocolate chips.
- Drop by teaspoonful onto ungreased cookie sheet.
- Bake until light brown, 8 to 10 minutes. Immediately remove from pan.
- Cool. Yield: About 4 dozen small cookies.

299.   Pumpkin Pie Squares Recipe

Serving: 9 | Prep: | Cook: 40mins | Ready in:

Ingredients

- Base Ingredients:
- 3/4 cup flour
- 1/2 cup rolled oats
- 1/4 cup brown sugar, packed
- 1/2 cup butter
- 1/2 cup chopped pecans
- ....
- Topping:
- One 14-ounce can of pumpkin
- One 10-ounce can of Eagle Brand sweetened condensed milk
- 2 eggs, beaten
- 1 teaspoon ginger
- 1 teaspoon cinnamon
- 1/2 cup coconut

Direction

- Base: mix base ingredients and press into a 9-inch square pan. Bake at 350 degrees for 15 minutes.
- Topping:
- In a separate bowl, mix topping ingredients except for coconut. Pour over base and bake at 350 degrees for 25 to 30 minutes or until set. Add coconut for topping. Serve with whipped cream.

300.   Pumpkin Spice Cookie Recipe

Serving: 60 | Prep: | Cook: 12mins | Ready in:

Ingredients

- 2 1/2 cups all-purpose flour
- 1 teaspoon baking powder

- 1 teaspoon baking soda
- 2 teaspoons ground cinnamon
- 1/2 teaspoon ground nutmeg
- 1/2 teaspoon ground cloves
- 1/2 teaspoon salt
- 1/2 cup butter, softened
- 1 1/2 cups white sugar
- 1 cup canned pumpkin puree
- 1 egg
- 1 teaspoon vanilla extract
- Frosting:
- 2 cups confectioners' sugar
- 3 tablespoons milk
- 1 tablespoon melted butter
- 1 teaspoon vanilla extract

Direction

- Preheat oven to 350 degrees F (175 degrees C).
- Combine flour, baking powder, baking soda, cinnamon, nutmeg, ground cloves, and salt; set aside.
- In a medium bowl, cream together the 1/2 cup of butter and white sugar.
- Add pumpkin, egg, and 1 teaspoon vanilla to butter mixture, and beat until creamy.
- Mix in dry ingredients.
- Drop on cookie sheet by tablespoonfuls; flatten slightly.
- Bake for 15 to 20 minutes in the preheated oven.
- Cool cookies, then drizzle glaze with fork.
- To Make Glaze:
- Combine confectioners' sugar, milk, 1 tablespoon melted butter, and 1 teaspoon vanilla. Add milk as needed, to achieve drizzling consistency.

301.   Pumpkin Squares Recipe

Serving: 12 | Prep: | Cook: 60mins | Ready in:

Ingredients

- Crust ~

- 1 c. flour
- 1/2 c. quick cooking oats
- 1/2 c. packed brown sugar
- 1/2 c. softened unsalted butter
- Filling ~
- 1 15 oz. can 100% pure pumpkin
- 1 12 oz. can evaporated milk
- 1/2 c. sugar
- 2 lg. eggs (or substitute)
- 1 t. ground cinnamon
- 1/2 t. salt
- 1/2 t. ground ginger
- 1/4 t. ground cloves
- Topping ~
- 1/4 c. packed brown sugar
- 1/2 c. chopped pecans or walnuts

Direction

- Preheat oven to 350.
- For Crust ~
- Beat flour, oats, brown sugar & butter in small mixer until crumbly.
- Press on to bottom of ungreased 13 x 9" baking pan.
- Bake for 15 minutes.
- For Filling ~
- Beat pumpkin, milk, sugar, eggs, spices, salt in large bowl until smooth.
- Pour over crust and bake for additional 20 minutes.
- For Topping ~
- Combine brown sugar & nuts in small bowl & sprinkle over filling.
- Bake for additional 15 to 25 minutes or till knife inserted in center comes out clean.
- Cool completely in pan on wire rack.
- Refrigerate until ready to serve.
- Top with whipped cream, if desired.

302.   Puzzle Pieces Recipe

Serving: 24 | Prep: | Cook: 10mins | Ready in:

Ingredients

- 1 stick butter
- 1 stick margarine
- 1/2 cup granulated sugar
- 1/2 box graham crackers
- 3/4 cup broken pecans

Direction

- Line a large cookie sheet with graham crackers.
- Melt butter and margarine in a saucepan.
- Stir in sugar and bring to a boil and pour over graham crackers.
- Sprinkle broken pecans over top and bake at 350 for 10 minutes.
- Remove from cookies sheet quickly because they set up pretty fast.
- Cool completely on a wire rack.

303.   Quick And Easy Cookies Recipe

Serving: 24 | Prep: | Cook: 10mins | Ready in:

Ingredients

- Any flavor cake mix.
- 2 eggs
- 1/2 cup vegetable oil
- Optional - Add nuts, chocolate chips, or anything else you think might be good.

Direction

- Mix all ingredients.
- Heat oven to 350 degrees.
- Drop spoonful of dough on ungreased cookie sheet 1-2 inches apart depending on the size of your cookies.
- Cook for 8 to 10 minutes (or a little more for large cookies).
- Refrigerate leftover dough for tomorrow.

- I used German Chocolate cake mix and added pecans and milk chocolate chips. I am going to try Spice Cake next.

304.   Quick And Easy Nutty Cheese Bars Recipe

Serving: 36 | Prep: | Cook: 25mins | Ready in:

Ingredients

- 1 butter pecan cake mix
- 3/4 cup margarine, melted
- 1 1/2 cups chopped pecans
- 1 cup brown sugar, packed
- 2 8-oz pkgs. cream cheese, softened

Direction

- Preheat oven to 350 degrees and grease a 9x13 pan.
- Stir together cake mix, margarine and HALF the pecans.
- Press mixture evenly into pan.
- Beat brown sugar and cream cheese together until well mixed.
- Spread over base.
- Sprinkle remaining pecans over top and gently pat into cheese.
- Bake 25-30 minutes until edges are browned.
- Cool and store in closed container in fridge.

305.   Raisin Banana Energy Bars Recipe

Serving: 24 | Prep: | Cook: 20mins | Ready in:

Ingredients

- 2 cups quick cooking oats
- 1 cup chopped nuts
- 1/3 cup butter

- 1/2 cup firmly packed brown sugar
- 1/4 cup honey
- 1 cup raisins
- 1 cup dried banana chips
- 1 cup honey coated graham cereal squares

Direction

- Heat oven to 350° then in square pan combine oats and nuts.
- Bake 20 minutes or until oats are toasted golden brown stirring occasionally.
- Meanwhile combine butter, brown sugar and honey in small saucepan.
- Cook over medium heat until mixture boils then pour over oat mixture.
- Add raisins, banana chips and cereal squares then toss to coat.
- With lightly floured hands press firmly into pan then bake at 350° for 10 minutes.
- Cool completely then cut into bars.

306. Raspberry And Almond Squares Recipe

Serving: 8 | Prep: | Cook: 60mins | Ready in:

Ingredients

- 9 oz chopped butter
- 9 oz self-raisin flour
- 5 oz ground almonds
- 5 oz light muscovado sugar
- 12 oz raspberries, fresh or frozen
- 3 oz caster sugar, plus extra
- 2 oz flaked almonds

Direction

- Preheat the oven and line a baking tin with baking parchment.
- Rub the butter into the flour, almonds and muscovado sugar to make crumbs, then firmly press 2 thirds onto the base and sides of the

tin. Toss the raspberries with the caster sugar, then scatter over the top.
- Mix the flaked almonds into the remaining crumbs, then scatter over the raspberries. Bake for 50-60 min until golden and the fruit is bubbling a little round the edges.
- Dredge with caster sugar, then cool in the tin.
- Cut into about 8 squares and enjoy with a cup of tea, coffee... or serve as a dessert with ice-cream or custard.

307. Red Plum Crumb Bars Recipe

Serving: 24 | Prep: | Cook: 25mins | Ready in:

Ingredients

- 1 cup brown sugar firmly packed
- 1-1/2 cups flour
- 3/4 cup butter
- 1-1/2 cups oatmeal
- 1/2 teaspoon baking soda
- 1 teaspoon vanilla extract
- 1/2 teaspoon salt
- 2 cups red plum jam
- powdered sugar

Direction

- Mix all ingredients except jam until crumbly.
- Spread 1/2 of the mixture into a greased rectangular pan.
- Spread jam over crumbly mixture then cover with remaining crumbs.
- Bake at 350° for 25 minutes then allow to cool 5 minutes.
- Sprinkle with powdered sugar.

308.   Reese's Peanut Butter Rice Crispies Cookies Recipe

Serving: 0 | Prep: | Cook: 12mins | Ready in:

Ingredients

- 1 cup (2 sticks) butter or margarine, softened
- 2 cups sugar
- 3 cups all purpose flour
- 1 teaspoon baking soda
- 1 teaspoon baking powder
- 1/2 teaspoon salt
- 2 to 3 eggs
- 4 cups rice crispies
- 2 packages (10 oz) peanut butter chips

Direction

- 1. Preheat oven to 3530 degrees. Lightly spray 2 cookie sheets.
- 2. Cream together butter and sugar with a mixer till well blended. Add the flour, baking soda, baking powder and salt and mix well. Beat in vanilla and eggs
- 3. Add the cereal and peanut butter chips and mix well with a spoon.
- 4. Drop cookies by spoonfuls 1 to 2 inches apart. Bake for 10 to 12 minutes or till golden or however you like them. Let them cool for 1 to 2 minutes than transfer to a metal rack to cool the rest of the way.

309.   Reeses Peanut Butter Cookies Recipe

Serving: 0 | Prep: | Cook: 25mins | Ready in:

Ingredients

- 2 cups all purpose flour
- 1/2 tsp baking soda
- 1/4 tsp salt
- 1 cup brown sugar
- 1 cup granulated sugar
- 1 cup butter, softened
- 3 eggs
- 1 cup peanut butter
- 2 tsp vanilla extract
- 1 1/2 cups reeses peanut butter baking chips

Direction

- Preheat oven to 300 degrees F (150 degrees C).
- In a medium bowl, combine flour, soda, and salt. Mix well with a wire whisk set aside.
- In a large bowl, blend sugars, using an electric mixer set at medium speed. Add butter, and mix to form a grainy paste, scraping the sides of the bowl. Add eggs, peanut butter and vanilla and mix at medium speed until light and fluffy.
- Add the flour mixture and mix at low speed until just mixed. Add baking chips and mix until incorporated.
- Drop by rounded spoonful onto an ungreased cookie sheet. Bake for 18-22 minutes or until slightly brown along edges. 18 minutes is perfect in my oven.
- Allow to cool on baking sheet about 2 minutes before placing on cooling rack.

310.   Relistic Peach Cookies Recipe

Serving: 24 | Prep: | Cook: 20mins | Ready in:

Ingredients

- 3/4 cup unsalted butter
- 1 cup white sugar
- 2 eggs
- 1 teaspoon vanilla extract
- 3 3/4 cups all-purpose flour
- 1 teaspoon baking powder
- 1/2 cup milk
- *
- 1/4 cup semisweet chocolate chips
- 2/3 cup apricot jam
- 1/3 cup ground pecans

- 2 teaspoons rum
- *
- 1/4 cup water
- 1 cup white sugar
- 2 drops red food coloring
- 4 drops yellow food coloring

Direction

- Preheat the oven to 325 degrees F (165 degrees C).
- Cream together the butter and 1 cup sugar until smooth.
- Beat in the eggs, one at a time
- Stir in the vanilla.
- In a separate bowl combine the flour and baking powder
- Stir into the creamed mixture alternately with the milk.
- Roll dough into 1-inch balls and place balls 1 inch apart onto an ungreased cookie sheet.
- Bake for 15 to 20 minutes in the preheated oven, until cookies start to brown on the bottom. Remove from baking sheets and cool on wire racks.
- When cookies are completely cool, carve a hole into the flat side of each cookie using a small knife
- Save the crumbs. In a heatproof bowl, melt chocolate chips
- Stir frequently until smooth
- In a medium bowl, stir together the melted chocolate, apricot jam, ground pecans, rum and reserved crumbs until well blended.
- Fill the carved-out centers of the cookies with the chocolate mixture and stick two cookies together with the filling sides in to form a peach shape.
- Divide the remaining cup of sugar into two bowls.
- One bowl should contain 1/4 cup and 3/4 cup in the other.
- Color the small bowl with the red coloring by working it in with your fingers.
- Color the other bowl with the yellow coloring and add a pinch of the red sugar to it to make a peachy color.

- Brush each cookie with water and roll them first in the yellow sugar, then dip a part of them into the red sugar to give them a blush. Insert angelica stems into the top for a realistic effect.

---

311. Rice Krispies Ice Cream Bars Recipe

Serving: 1 | Prep: | Cook: | Ready in:

Ingredients

- 3 cups crushed Rice Krispies
- 1 cup grated coconut
- 3/4 cup finely chopped pecans
- 1/2 cup brown sugar, firmly packed
- 1/2 cup butter, melted
- 1/2 gallon vanilla ice cream
- Topping (your choice)

Direction

- Combine Rice Krispies, coconut, pecans, sugar and butter. Spread half of the mixture on the bottom of a 9 x 13-inch cake pan. Pat into place.
- Slice vanilla ice cream and place on top of mixture. Spread other half of Rice Krispies mixture on top. Freeze.
- To serve, slice into bars and serve with chocolate syrup or other topping of choice

---

312. Rich Chocolate Pumpkin Truffles Recipe

Serving: 48 | Prep: | Cook: 25mins | Ready in:

Ingredients

- 2-1/2 cups (about 62) crushed vanilla wafers
- 1 cup ground almonds, toasted

- 3/4 cup sifted powdered sugar, divided
- 2 teaspoons ground cinnamon
- 1 cup (6 ounces) NESTLE® TOLL HOUSE® Semi-sweet chocolate Morsels, melted (follow melting direction on NESTLE package)
- 1/2 cup LIBBY'S 100% Pure pumpkin
- 1/3 cup coffee liqueur or apple juice

Direction

- COMBINE crushed cookies, ground almonds, 1/2 cup powdered sugar and cinnamon in medium bowl.
- Blend in melted chocolate, pumpkin, and coffee liqueur.
- Shape into 1-inch balls. Chill.
- Dust with remaining powdered sugar just before serving.

---

313.   Rolo Chocolate Cookies Recipe

Serving: 48 | Prep: | Cook: 10mins | Ready in:

Ingredients

- 2-1/4 cups flour
- 3/4 cup unsweetened cocoa
- 1 tsp. baking soda
- 1 cup sugar
- 1 cup firmly packed brown sugar
- 1 cup butter or margarine, softened
- 2 tsps. vanilla
- 2 eggs
- 1 cup chopped pecans
- 48 Rolo caramels, unwrapped (9-oz. pkg.)
- Heat oven to 325. Lightly spoon flour into measuring cup; level off .

Direction

- Heat oven to 325. Lightly spoon flour into measuring cup; level off. In small bowl, combine flour, baking soda and cocoa; blend well.

- *In large bowl, beat 1 cup sugar, brown sugar, and margarine until light and fluffy. Add vanilla and eggs; beat well. Add flour mixture; blend well. Stir in 1/2 cup of the pecans Chill dough for a little while to stiffen. For each cookie, with floured hands, shape about 1 tablespoonful dough around 1 caramel candy, covering completely.
- In small bowl, combine remaining 1/2 cup pecans and 1 TBSP sugar. Press one side of each ball into pecan mixture. Place, nut side up, 2 inches apart on ungreased cookie sheets.
- Bake at 325 for 10 minutes or until set and slightly cracked. Cool 2 minutes; remove from cookie sheets. Cool completely on wire rack.

---

314.   Russian Tea Cakes Recipe

Serving: 10 | Prep: | Cook: 15mins | Ready in:

Ingredients

- 1 cup butter, soft
- 1/2 cup confectioners' sugar
- 1 teaspoon vanilla
- 2 1/4 cups all-purpose flour, sifted
- 1/4 teaspoon salt
- 1/3 cup finely chopped nuts

Direction

- Preheat oven to 400 degrees F.
- Grease a cookie sheet.
- Cream together the butter, sugar and vanilla.
- Sift flour.
- Resift flour with the salt.
- Stir flour mixture into butter mixture.
- Mix well.
- Stir in the chopped nuts.
- Form dough into 1" balls.
- Placed on prepared cookie sheet.
- Bake 14 to 17 minutes.
- Roll in confectioners' sugar.

315. SWEETHEART MELTS Recipe

Serving: 1 | Prep: | Cook: 10mins | Ready in:

Ingredients

- 2 slices white bread
- melted butter
- peanut butter
- you favorite candy bar, broken into pieces (or chocolate chips)
- mini marshmallows
- powdered sugar, cinnamon sugar or colored sugar

Direction

- Trim the edges from the bread and cut each slice into a large heart shape. Brush one side of each heart with melted butter. Place one heart, butter side down, in a skillet. Spread peanut butter on top. Place the candy bar pieces on the peanut butter and sprinkle with mini marshmallows. Top with the other heart, butter side up. Cook slowly until the chocolate is melted and the hearts are nicely browned on both sides. Before serving, dust with powdered sugar, cinnamon sugar or colored sugar.

316. Saiyges Super Evil Oatmeal Cookies Of Doom Recipe

Serving: 1 | Prep: | Cook: 13mins | Ready in:

Ingredients

- 1/2 cup applesauce
- 1/2 cup butter
- 1 tsp. vanilla
- 2 eggs
- 1/2 cup brown sugar
- 1/2 cup sugar
- 1/2 tsp. cinnamon
- 1/8 tsp. clove
- 1 tsp. baking soda
- 1 tsp. salt
- 2 cups flour
- 3 1/2 cups quick cooking oats
- 1/2 cup chopped pecans
- 1/2 cup semi-sweet chocolate chip morsels
- ****Substitutions! - You CAN!!!! replace -all- of the butter with an extra 1/2c. of applesauce - or- replace the applesauce with 1c. puree pumpkin (not pumpkin pie mix, just the puree... the stuff without all the extra gunk added!) The cookies come out slightly more cakelike, and you may want to add a little more oats/flour.

Direction

- Cream together butter, white sugar, brown sugar, and vanilla.
- Add in eggs and applesauce until blended.
- Mix in Cinnamon, Clove, salt and baking soda.
- Add flour until blended, then oats.
- When this is all mixed, add pecans and chocolate chips.
- Drop by the spoonful onto ungreased cookie sheets and bake at 375 F for 15 minutes.
- GENTLY remove cookies from cookie sheets onto a rack and allow to cool for at -least- five minutes. I'm serious. I mean it. You let them cool! Arm yourself with a wooden spoon.... you might need to threaten family members, significant others, roommates and random innocent people just passing by who lose all sense of self control near these cookies.
- Don't say I didn't warn you.

317. Samoa Bars Recipe

Serving: 30 | Prep: | Cook: 2hours25mins | Ready in:

Ingredients

- COOKIE BASE
- 1 1/2 cups sugar
- 3/4 cup butter, softened
- 1 large egg
- 1/2 teaspoon vanilla extract
- 2 cups all-purpose flour
- 1 1/2 tsp. salt
- TOPPING
- 3 cups shredded coconut, toasted
- 1 (14oz) bag caramels
- 1/2 teaspoon salt
- 3 tablespoons milk
- 10 oz simi-sweet chocolate (chocolate chips ok)

Direction

- Preheat oven to 350°F
- For the cookie base
- Line a 9×13-inch baking pan with aluminum foil, and spray it lightly with cooking spray.
- In a large bowl, cream together sugar and butter, until fluffy.
- Beat in egg and vanilla extract.
- Working at a low speed, gradually beat in flour and salt until mixture is crumbly, like wet sand.
- Pour crumbly dough into prepared pan and press into an even layer.
- Bake for 20-25 minutes, until base is set and edges are lightly browned.
- Cool completely on a wire rack.
- For the topping
- Unwrap the caramels and place in a large microwave-safe bowl with milk and salt.
- Microwave on high for 3-4 minutes, stopping to stir a few times to help the caramel melt.
- When smooth, fold in toasted coconut with a spatula.
- Put dollops of the topping all over the shortbread base.
- Using the spatula, spread the topping in an even layer.
- Let topping set until cooled. When cooled, cut into 30 bars with a large knife or a pizza cutter.

- Once bars are cut, melt chocolate in a small bowl. Heat it on high in the microwave in 45-second intervals, stirring thoroughly to prevent scorching.
- Dip the base of each bar into the chocolate and place on a clean piece of wax paper.
- Use remaining chocolate (or melt a bit of additional chocolate, if necessary) to drizzle bars with chocolate to finish. Let chocolate set completely before storing in an airtight container.

318. Scary Oreo Spiders Recipe

Serving: 0 | Prep: | Cook: |Ready in:

Ingredients

- 25g pack Halloween Mini Oreos (approx 7 in each bag)
- 7 black liquorice bootlaces (each cut into four equal sized pieces)
- 1 tube of pre-prepared white chocolate flavoured icing (7 grams, two dots, per spider)

Direction

- Using a kitchen scissors, cut the liquor ice bootlace into eight legs.
- Insert 4 pieces of strawberry liquor ice bootlace into either side of each Mini Oreo.
- Using ready-prepared decorating icing, pipe 2 small dots for eyes on each Mini Oreo.

319. Scrumptious Chocolate Layer Bars Recipe

Serving: 36 | Prep: | Cook: 35mins |Ready in:

Ingredients

- Filling:

- 12 oz chocolate chips
- 5 oz Can evaporated milk
- 8 oz cream cheese
- 1/2 ts almond extract
- Crust:
- 3 c flour
- 1 c butter, softened
- 2 eggs
- 1 ts baking powder
- 1/2 ts almond extract

Direction

- Mix chocolate chips, cream cheese and evaporated milk in a saucepan. Cook over low heat, stirring constantly, until mixture is smooth. Remove from heat and stir in 1/2 tsp. almond extract. Mix well; set aside.
- Combine remaining ingredients. Blend well until mixture resembles coarse crumbs.
- Press 1/2 crumbs (not too hard) in greased 9 x 13 pan. Spread with chocolate mixture. Sprinkle remaining 1/2 of crumbs over filling.
- Bake at 375 degrees F for 35-40 minutes or until golden brown. Cool and cut into bars. Makes approx. 36 bars.

320.   Shrewsbury Biscuits Recipe

Serving: 6 | Prep: | Cook: 30mins | Ready in:

Ingredients

- 250 gms butter
- 300 gms caster sugar
- 3-4 egg yolks
- 450 gms flour
- Grated rind of two lemons

Direction

- Strain the flour through a fine mesh twice.

- Cream the butter and sugar with a whisk until the yellow of the butter becomes off white and the mixture is fluffy.
- Beat the egg yolks till runny, add to the butter mixture and mix well.
- Add the flour and grated lemon rind and stir in with a spoon till it makes a firm but not stiff dough.
- Flour a surface and knead the dough gently for a minute or so. Roll out to 1/4" thick. Using a cookie cutter cut out circles of 2 diameter.
- Place on a greased and floured baking sheet. Bake at Mark 4 or 350 degrees F for about 15 minutes till very lightly browned.
- Let it cool down completely and then store in an air tight jar
- Enjoy!!!!
- Tip:
- Last time when I made it I was running out of lemon so I found vanilla sugar with lemon flavour. It turned out well only the taste changed a little. You can change or add more ingredients as per your choice.

321.   Simple Peanut Butter Cookies Recipe

Serving: 60 | Prep: | Cook: 10mins | Ready in:

Ingredients

- 1 cup unsalted butter, softened
- 1 cup crunchy peanut butter (can use creamy)
- 1 cup granulated sugar
- 1 cup light brown sugar, slightly packed
- 2 eggs
- 2 1/2 cups all purpose flour
- 1 tsp. baking powder
- 1 1/2 tsp. baking soda
- 1/2 tsp. salt

Direction

- Preheat oven to 375 degrees. 350 degrees if using a dark pan.

- Cream together butter, peanut butter, eggs, and sugars.
- In a separate bowl, sift together flour, baking soda, baking powder, and salt.
- Stir into batter.
- Refrigerate for an hour.
- Roll into 1" balls. Put on cookie evenly spaced.
- Flatten with for in a crisscross.
- Bake at 375 degrees for about 10 minutes.

322. Smores Bars Recipe

Serving: 24 | Prep: | Cook: 25mins | Ready in:

Ingredients

- 3/4 cup butter
- 2/3 cup sugar
- 1 egg
- 1 teaspoon vanilla
- 18 whole graham crackers, crushed (approx 3 cups)
- 1/2 cup all-purpose flour
- 1/2 teaspoon salt
- 8 milk chocolate bars - 1 1/2 oz each
- 3 1/2 cups miniature marshmallows

Direction

- Heat oven to 350°.
- Beat butter and sugar with electric mixer on medium speed until light and fluffy.
- Beat in egg and vanilla.
- Stir in crushed graham crackers, flour, and salt. Reserve 1 cup of the graham cracker mixture and press remaining mixture over the bottom of a greased 13x9x2-inch baking pan.
- Arrange chocolate bars, in a single layer, over graham cracker crust mixture in the pan.
- Sprinkle with marshmallows.
- Crumbled reserved graham cracker mixture over the marshmallows.
- Bake for 20 to 25 minutes or until golden brown.
- Cool in pan on wire rack for 10 minutes.

- Cut into bars and cool completely.
- Makes about 2 dozen bars.

323. Snappy Gingersnaps Recipe

Serving: 0 | Prep: | Cook: 60mins | Ready in:

Ingredients

- 2-1/4 C. all-purpose flour
- 2 tsps. baking soda
- 1 tsp. ginger
- 1 tsp. cinnamon
- 1/2 tsp. cloves
- 1/4 tsp. salt
- 3/4 C. butter-flavored shortening (I use Crisco sticks for convenience)
- 1/2 C. granulated sugar
- 1/2 C. packed brown sugar
- 1 large egg
- 1/4 C. molasses
- 1/4 C. chopped crystallized ginger, or to taste (optional)
- Granulated sugar

Direction

- Heat oven to 350 degrees. In a large bowl, whisk together flour, baking soda, ginger, cinnamon, cloves, and salt; set aside. In another large bowl, cream together shortening, granulated sugar, and brown sugar. Add egg and molasses and mix well. Gradually stir in flour mixture just until combined. Stir in crystallized ginger, if using. Shape dough into 1-inch balls. Roll balls in granulated sugar and place on greased or parchment paper lined baking sheet. Bake 8-9 mins. or until cookies are set and the tops are cracked (see note). Cool a few mins. on baking sheet. Remove cookies to a wire rack and cool completely.
- Note: The above bake time results in a soft, chewy cookie, just the way we like 'em! If you prefer crisp, crunchy cookies, bake longer.

Recipe is easily doubled and the cookies freeze well.

324. Snicker Filled Peanut Butter Cookies Recipe

Serving: 1 | Prep: | Cook: 13mins | Ready in:

Ingredients

- 1/2 cup granulated sugar
- 1/2 cup brown sugar
- 1/2 cup butter, softened
- 1 egg
- 1/2 cup peanut butter
- 1/4 teaspoon salt
- 1 1/2 cups all-purpose flour
- 1/2 teaspoon baking powder
- 1/2 teaspoon baking soda
- 20 fun-sized Snicker candy bars **

Direction

- Mix all together except candy bars. Shape dough around each candy piece
- Place 4 inches apart on ungreased cookie sheet. Bake at 350 degrees F for 13-15 minutes
- Cool for 10 minutes.
- ** Note: I cut the fun sized Snicker bars into thirds....or you could use the bite-size Snickers.

325. Snow Balls Recipe

Serving: 24 | Prep: | Cook: 10mins | Ready in:

Ingredients

- 1 cup butter (softened)
- 3/4 cup sugar
- 2 cups flour
- 8 oz package Hershey kisses
- powder sugar

Direction

- Preheat oven at 350 degrees. Cream butter and sugar until smooth. Add flour to the mixture and completely blend. Wrap in plastic wrap and place in frig for 30 minutes. Remove foil from Hershey kisses. Remove dough from frig and shape into 1-inch balls - inserting a kiss in center of each ball (make sure it is completely covered by the dough). Bake on ungreased cookie sheet for 10 minutes. Place powdered sugar in a small bowl and one by one put a cookie in while they are still warm, and roll them around a bit to coat them with sugar. Let cool completely before serving as the kiss inside can stay very hot for a while.

326. Snowball Cookies Recipe

Serving: 6 | Prep: | Cook: 20mins | Ready in:

Ingredients

- 2c. flour
- 1/2t. salt
- 3/4c butter
- 1/2c sugar
- 2t. vanilla
- 1 egg
- 1(6oz.) pkg. chocolate chips
- confectioners sugar

Direction

- Use mixer to cream butter, sugar, vanilla and egg: stir in flour and salt.
- Add chocolate chips. Shape into balls 1" round. Bake on ungreased cookie sheet for 15-20 mins. at 350. Roll in confectioners' sugar

327. Snowballs Recipe

Serving: 36 | Prep: | Cook: | Ready in:

Ingredients

- 2 3/4 c vanilla wafers, crushed fine
- 1 c powdered sugar, sifted
- 1/4 c butter, melted
- 1/4 c frozen orange juice concentrate
- Extra powdered sugar

Direction

- Combine wafers & 1 c powdered sugar.
- Add butter & oj concentrate.
- Mix well, adding a bit more concentrate if too dry.
- Roll in small balls.
- Roll balls in powdered sugar.
- Refrigerate a few hours till balls are firm.
- Flavors really come to life the longer they sit.
- Freeze & thaw well for later use.

---

328.   Soda Cracker Cookies Recipe

Serving: 10 | Prep: | Cook: 9mins | Ready in:

Ingredients

- soda crackers
- ½ cup sugar
- 1 cup (2 sticks) butter or margarine
- 12 oz. chocolate chips
- 1 ½ cups chopped nuts (optional)

Direction

- Preheat oven to 325°F.
- Line jelly roll pan (aka cookie sheet) with foil, overlapping the sides.
- Line pan with soda crackers (saltines) in a single layer, to cover pan.
- Stir and boil together sugar and butter in a small saucepan for 3 minutes.
- Pour sugar/butter mixture over crackers and spread evenly.

- Bake for approximately 8 minutes...it will be golden and bubbly but not brown.
- As soon as it is out of the oven, sprinkle approximately 12 ounces of chocolate chips on top of the crackers.
- Put pan back in oven for about 1 minute to help chocolate melt.
- Remove and spread chocolate with a knife.
- Sprinkle 1 ½ cup chopped nuts on top of chocolate, covering all.
- Press slightly so nuts adhere to chocolate.
- Put pan in freezer and cool for approximately 30 minutes.
- Peel back foil gently from cookies and break cookies into pieces. Keeps best in a covered container in the refrigerator.
- (I use pecans... I roast them in the oven for about 5 minutes for optimal flavor, then finely chop them.)
- These are really good and unusual... easy, too! I wouldn't use margarine unless I had no choice.
- Number of servings really vary.

---

329.   Soft Spice Bars Recipe

Serving: 0 | Prep: | Cook: 10mins | Ready in:

Ingredients

- 3/4 cup butter, melted
- 1 cup plus 2 tbsp sugar, divided
- 1/4 cup molasses
- 1 egg
- 2 cups flour
- 2 tsp baking soda
- 1 tsp ground cinnamon
- 1/2 tsp salt
- 1/2 tsp ground ginger
- 1/2 tsp ground cloves

Direction

- In a large mixing bowl, combine the butter, 1 cup of the sugar, and the molasses

- Beat in the egg until smooth
- Combine the flour, baking soda, cinnamon, salt, ginger, and cloves
- Stir into the molasses mixture
- Spread into a greased 15 x 10 inch baking pan
- Sprinkle with the remaining sugar
- Bake at 375 F for 10-12 minutes or until lightly browned (Do Not Overbake)
- Cool on a wire rack
- Cut into bars

330. Sour Cream Cranberry Bars Recipe

Serving: 16 | Prep: | Cook: 40mins | Ready in:

Ingredients

- 1 cup packed brown sugar
- 1 cup butter softened
- 2 cups quick cooking oats
- 1-1/2 cups cake flour
- 1 teaspoon baking soda
- 2 cups sweetened dried cranberries
- 1 cup sour cream
- 3/4 cup sugar
- 2 tablespoons cake flour
- 1 tablespoon grated lemon peel
- 1 teaspoon vanilla
- 1 egg

Direction

- Preheat oven to 350 then mix brown sugar and butter in large bowl with spoon.
- Stir in oats, flour and baking soda until crumbly.
- Press half of the mixture in bottom of ungreased rectangular pan and bake 10 minutes.
- Mix remaining ingredients in large bowl and pour over baked crust.
- Crumble remaining oats over filling and bake 30 minutes longer then cool completely.

331. Special K Bar Cookies Recipe

Serving: 24 | Prep: | Cook: 10mins | Ready in:

Ingredients

- Special K Bar cookies
- 1 1/2 C. sugar
- 1 1/2 C. peanut butter (Creamy or Crunchy)
- 1 1/2 C. white corn syrup
- 1 t. maple flavoring
- 1 Box Special K cereal (the Large size)
- Topping:
- 1 1/2 C. butterscotch chips
- 1 1/2 C. chocolate chips
- Add maple flavoring to taste -- as well as vanilla flavoring
- Mix above together and bring to a boil in pan allowing to boil for a couple minutes- stirring occassionally. Gradually add Special

Direction

- Bring sugar, peanut butter, corn syrup and maple flavoring to boil-- boil a couple minutes. Gradually add the cereal to the melted mixture.
- Spread out in a 9X13 pan.
- Prepare topping. Melt butterscotch chips, chocolate chips and flavorings together and spread over the cereal mixture in pan. Let cool, cut and serve.
- You can vary ingredients in order to create a very gooey bar cookie and if you prefer-- you may refrigerate the cookies.
- Super easy recipe, kids love them!

332. Stumps Nut Butter Balls Recipe

Serving: 8 | Prep: | Cook: 15mins | Ready in:

Ingredients

- 1c soft butter
- 2c sifted flour
- 1/2tsp salt
- 1/4-1/2c powdered sugar
- 2tsp vanilla OR
- 1tsp almond extract
- 1-2c finely chopped nuts

Direction

- Mix butter with sugar until creamy.
- Add salt, extract, flour, nuts: mix well.
- Chill dough until easy to handle.
- Heat oven to 350 degrees.
- Using fingers, shape dough into 1"balls or 2 " rolls.
- Place on ungreased cookie sheet.
- Bake 12-15 minutes until light brown.
- While cookies are warm roll them in powdered sugar.

333. Stumps Peanut Butter Cookies Recipe

Serving: 8 | Prep: | Cook: 15mins | Ready in:

Ingredients

- 2 1/2c flour
- 1c butter or margarine
- 1c peanut butter
- 1c white sugar
- 1c brown sugar
- 2 eggs beaten
- 1tsp baking soda
- 1/2tsp salt

Direction

- Cream butter with sugar.
- Next add peanut butter.
- Add eggs then the rest of the ingredients.
- Chill several hours.
- Form into balls the size of small walnuts.
- Place on greased cookie sheet.
- Flatten balls slightly with the bottom of a fork horizontally and vertically.
- Bake in "quick oven" at 350 degrees until light brown.

334. Sues Butter Balls Recipe

Serving: 48 | Prep: | Cook: 18mins | Ready in:

Ingredients

- 1 cup butter
- 4 Tbsp. powdered sugar
- 1 tsp. vanilla
- 2 cups flour
- 1 cup finely chopped pecans

Direction

- I mix all with hands, roll into small balls. Bake at 350 for 18 min. Let cool. Roll in powdered sugar.

335. Sugar Free Chocolate Tea Cookies Recipe

Serving: 24 | Prep: | Cook: 20mins | Ready in:

Ingredients

- 1/4 cup butter
- 3 tablespoons Splenda (more to taste if desired)
- 2 eggs
- 1/2 teaspoon vanilla extract
- 2 tablespoon milk (whole or skim)

- 1 1/4 cups cake flour
- 1 ounce square of unsweetened bakers chocolate (melted)

Direction

- Cream butter. Add Splenda, eggs, vanilla extract and milk. Blend well.
- Add half of the flour, mix well and stir in the melted chocolate.
- Add the rest of the flour and mix well.
- Flour your hands and roll dough into small balls. Press each ball with your finger to flatten on an ungreased cookie sheet.
- Bake in a preheated oven at 350 degrees F (175 degrees C) for 20 minutes.
- Remove from the oven and set each cookie of a wire rack to cool.

---

336. Super Easy Walnut Spice Bars Recipe

Serving: 20 | Prep: | Cook: 30mins | Ready in:

Ingredients

- 1 spice cake mix (I had Betty Crocker Super Moist)
- 1 stick butter
- 1 egg
- 1/3 cup milk (or half 'n' half)
- 1/2 cup chopped walnuts (more if using English walnuts, they're not as pungent as Black)
- THAT'S IT!

Direction

- Pre-heat oven to 350*F
- Stir softened butter (I whip it up well with the spoon before adding other ingredients) cake mix, milk, egg, and nuts together really good.
- Spread evenly into greased 9 x 13 baking pan
- Cook for 30 minutes or until toothpick comes out clean.

- Cool slightly and cut into squares the size of your choice.
- Enjoy.

---

337. Surprise Teacakes Recipe

Serving: 36 | Prep: | Cook: 15mins | Ready in:

Ingredients

- 2/3 cup sugar
- 1 cup butter, softened
- 1 egg
- 1/2 teasp. salt
- 1 teasp. vanilla or almond extract (or one of your choice) I use vanilla
- 2 1/4 cup flour
- centers:
- chocolate mint candy, large chocolate chip, candied cherries, gum drops, chocolate covered nuts, etc

Direction

- Beat at med speed: sugar, butter, egg, salt and the extract of choice until well mixed.
- Add flour and beat for 1 min.
- Put cookie dough around your choice of centers and roll into a ball. If dough feels too soft put in refrigerator for 1/2 hour or so.
- Bake at 350° for 15-18 mins on a lightly greased cookie sheet.
- When cool put in a bag and coat with confectionary sugar.
- Or drizzle with some melted semi-sweet chocolate.

---

338. Sweet Lemon Bars Recipe

Serving: 16 | Prep: | Cook: 42mins | Ready in:

Ingredients

- For the Crust
- Ingredients:
- 1 cup all-purpose flour
- 5 Tbs. margarine or butter melted
- ¼ cup confectioners' sugar
- 1 tsp. Minced lemon peel
- 2 Tbs. skim milk
- Ingredients:
- For topping
- 1 cup granulated sugar or sweetener substitute
- 3 Tbs. Fresh lemon juice
- 2 Tbs. all-purpose flour
- 1 large egg
- 2 egg whites
- ½ tsp. baking powder
- confectioners' sugar for garnish

Direction

- 1. Preheat oven to 350°. Spray an 8" square baking pan with vegetable cooking spray.
- 2. To prepare crust, in a medium bowl, combine flour, margarine, confectioners' sugar, and lemon peel. Mix well. Pour in milk, stirring, until dough can be gathered into a ball.
- 3. Pat dough evenly into bottom and 1/4" up the sides of prepared pan. Bake until crust is golden, about 20 minutes. Place pan on a wire rack and cool for 5 minutes.
- 4. To prepare the topping, in a medium bowl, combine sugar, lemon juice, flour, egg, egg whites, and baking powder. Mix well.
- 5. Pour topping over prepared crust. Bake until topping is set, about 20 to 25 minutes. Place on a wire rack and cool completely. Cut into 2-inch squares. Dust with confectioners' sugar.
- Tip: For best results, thoroughly chill them first. Cold bars are less likely to crumble.
- Per Serving: Calories 128, Carbohydrates 21, Protein 2, Sodium 28mg, Fat 4, Cholesterol 23mg

---

339. Swirled Mint Cookies Recipe

Serving: 36 | Prep: | Cook: 10mins | Ready in:

Ingredients

- 2 cups flour
- 1/2 teaspoon baking powder
- 1 cup butter
- 1 cup granulated sugar
- 1 egg
- 1 teaspoon vanilla extract
- 1/2 teaspoon peppermint extract
- 10 drops ed food coloring
- 10 drops green food coloring

Direction

- Combine flour and baking powder then beat butter until softened.
- Add sugar and beat until fluffy the add egg and extracts and beat again.
- Add flour mixture and beat until well mixed.
- Divide dough into thirds then stir red food coloring into one third green into another.
- Leave third batch plan then cover each and chill one hour.
- Roll each color into 1/2" diameter ropes then using one rope of each color and twist together.
- Slice twisted ropes into 1/4" pieces then place slices 2" apart on ungreased cookie sheet.
- Flatten to 1/4" thickness with bottom of a glass dipped in sugar.
- Bake at 375 for 8 minutes then remove and cool on racks.

---

340. The Perfect Peanut Butter Cookie Recipe

Serving: 4 | Prep: | Cook: 11mins | Ready in:

Ingredients

- 1 1/2 cups all-purpose flour
- 1/2 teaspoon baking powder
- 1/2 teaspoon baking soda
- 1/2 teaspoon salt
- 1 cup creamy or chunky peanut butter
- 1/2 cup (1 stick) butter or margarine, softened
- 1/2cup firmly packed light brown sugar
- 1/2 cup granulated sugar
- 1 large egg
- 1/2 teaspoon vanilla extract

Direction

- Preheat oven to 400 degrees
- In a medium bowl sift to combine flour, baking powder, baking soda and salt
- In a large bowl beat together peanut butter, butter, brown sugar, and granulated sugar until smooth.
- Add in egg and vanilla
- Combine flour mixture with peanut butter mixture, scrapping the sides of the bowl to insure batter is well blended.
- Cover bowl with plastic and place in frig for 20 minutes
- Using a teaspoon drop batter 1 inch apart on an ungreased cookie sheet.
- Using a fork make crisscross pattern flattening cookies slightly.
- Bake for 10 to 12 minutes per your oven

341.   Toffee Apple Cookies Recipe

Serving: 36 | Prep: | Cook: 12mins | Ready in:

Ingredients

- 1/2 cup shortening
- 1/3 cup brown sugar
- 2 (3/4 oz) packets apple cider drink mix
- 1 tbsp golden corn syrup
- 1/2 tsp vanilla
- 1/4 tsp concentrated apple flavouring (Lorann's brand is what I used), optional
- 1 egg
- 1/2 cup flour
- 1/2 cup spelt flour
- 3/4 tsp baking soda
- 1/4 tsp salt
- 1/2 cup toffee pieces (like Skor)

Direction

- Heat oven to 375°F, and line cookie sheets with parchment paper.
- In large bowl, beat shortening and sugar until fluffy.
- Beat in drink mix, corn syrup, flavourings and egg.
- Mix together flours, baking soda and salt.
- Beat into creamed mixture.
- Stir in toffee pieces.
- Bake 12 minutes and cook on wire racks.

342.   Toffee Bars Recipe

Serving: 90 | Prep: | Cook: 20mins | Ready in:

Ingredients

- 1 c. butter
- 1 c. brown sugar (I use light brown)
- 1 egg yolk
- 1 t. vanilla
- 2 c. all-purpose flour
- 1 6-oz. package semi-sweet chocolate chips (I use more like 3 c., or 10 oz.)
- 1 c. almond slivers, roasted

Direction

- Cream together butter and sugar until light.
- Add egg yolk, vanilla, and sifted flour, and beat until smooth, scraping the sides of the bowl.

- Line a jelly roll pan (10" x 15 ", 1" sides) with parchment paper, letting it hang over the sides.
- Using a piece of plastic wrap to keep the stuff from sticking to your hand, spread the dough evenly over the parchment paper.
- Bake at 350 ° for 15-20 minutes, or until lightly puffed and golden brown. Don't let it get too dark!!
- Sprinkle the chocolate chips over the surface and return the pan to the oven for a minute, which is all it will take to melt the chocolate.
- Spread the chocolate evenly over the surface, then sprinkle the almonds over the surface, accepting the uneven distribution as part of life.
- Let cool at room temperature until the chocolate is firm, then cut into small squares or rectangles. If you can remove the stuff from the pan before cutting it up, cutting is easier, but don't worry if you can't, because that makes more broken ones needing to be gotten rid of. Pre-nibble yield: depends on how big you cut them; I end up with something like 90 cookies.

343.   Toffee Topped Bars Recipe

Serving: 1 | Prep: | Cook: 35mins | Ready in:

Ingredients

- 2 cups firmly packed brown sugar
- 2 cups all-purpose flour
- 1/2 cup margarine, softened
- 1 tsp. baking powder
- 1/2 tsp. salt
- 1 tsp. vanilla extract
- 1 cup milk
- 1 egg
- 1 cup chocolate chips
- 1/2 cup chopped walnuts or pecans
- 1/4 cup unsweetened flaked coconut(optional)

Direction

- Preheat oven to 350 degrees. Lightly grease a 13 x 9 inch baking pan; set aside.
- In a large mixing bowl, mix together the brown sugar and flour. Using a pastry cutter or two knives, cut in the butter until mixture resembles coarse crumbs. Remove 1 cup of mixture and set aside. To mixture in large bowl, add baking powder and salt. Using a fork, lightly beat in vanilla, milk and egg. Continue beating until a smooth batter forms. Pour batter into prepared baking pan. In a small bowl, combine the chocolate chips and nuts. Fold in the coconut.
- Sprinkle reserved crumb mixture over top of batter in pan. Sprinkle with the chocolate chips and nuts. Using a long flat spatula, spread topping evenly over the top of the batter in pan.
- Bake bars for 35 minutes, or until a skewer inserted in center comes out clean. Transfer pan to a wire rack. Cool bars in pan completely before slicing. Using a serrated knife, cut into 24 bars. Store in airtight container for up to 5 days.

344.   Tootsie Rum Balls Recipe

Serving: 36 | Prep: | Cook: 5mins | Ready in:

Ingredients

- 1/2 C rum
- 2 T butter
- 5 1/2 oz. pkg. bite-size Tootsie rolls
- 1 pkg. (not whole box of) graham crackers, crushed
- 1 c. walnuts, chopped fine
- 1 C Powderd sugar

Direction

- Melt Tootsie Rolls, butter and rum over low heat.
- Add crackers and nuts.
- Remove from heat and cool till can easily be worked into balls.
- Roll into balls, then roll in powdered sugar.
- Store in airtight container.
- Of course, number of servings depend on the size you make them...I usually make a double batch...they don't last long!

345.   Ultimate Chocolate Chip Cookies Recipe

Serving: 0 | Prep: | Cook: 1hours | Ready in:

Ingredients

- 3/4 cup granulated sugar
- 3/4 cup packed brown sugar
- 1 cup butter or margarine, softened
- 1 egg
- 2 1/4 cups all-purpose flour
- 1 teaspoon baking soda
- 1/2 teaspoon salt
- 1 cup coarsely chopped nuts
- 1 package (12 ounces) semisweet chocolate chips (2 cups)

Direction

- 1. Heat oven to 375°F.
- 2. Mix sugars, butter and egg in large bowl. Stir in flour, baking soda and salt (dough will be stiff). Stir in nuts and chocolate chips.
- 3. Drop dough by rounded tablespoonfuls about 2 inches apart onto ungreased cookie sheet.
- 4. Bake 8 to 10 minutes or until light brown (centers will be soft). Cool slightly; remove from cookie sheet. Cool on wire rack.

346.   Vanilla Cinnamon Rice Krispie Squares Recipe

Serving: 12 | Prep: | Cook: 15mins | Ready in:

Ingredients

- 10 oz. large marshmallows
- 3 tbsp. butter
- 6 cups Rice Krispies
- 1 1/2 tsp. vanilla extract
- 1 - 2 tsp. cinnamon (depending on how strong you want the flavor)

Direction

- Use a bit of wax paper, crumple it up, and smear it in some butter for using to grease a pan about 12 x 8 inches. Make sure you get the sides.
- Melt butter in large saucepan or large pot over medium heat.
- Toss in marshmallows, and stir until melted. If you don't take care stirring, they'll burn, so watch out!
- Remove from heat and while stirring, add in the vanilla extract and cinnamon.
- Pour in the Rice Krispies and stir to mix it all up. It gets really sticky and messy, but try to coat the cereal as best as you can.
- Spoon mixture into pan, and press down with either the back of a greased spoon, or greasy fingers, and just let them cool!
- If you want to keep them longer, cover with wax paper, and keep them in the fridge.

347.   Vanilla Cookies Recipe

Serving: 18 | Prep: | Cook: 15mins | Ready in:

Ingredients

- 1/2 cup butter,soft
- 1/4 cup sugar,grind it
- 1 1/4 cup flour

- 1/2 tsp vanilla essence
- 1/2 tsp baking powder

Direction

- Preheat oven at 180 C.
- Beat butter and sugar until creamy.
- Add vanilla and baking powder and beat.
- Add flour, a tablespoon at a time and continue beating until you get a soft dough.
- Mix well and make 18 equal sized balls.
- Flat them with the palm of your hand.
- Place on a greased baking sheet .Dip a folk in water and press the top of each to mark the cookies.
- Bake on 180 C for 12-15 minutes till the edges of cookies turn golden.
- Leave on the cookie sheet for 2-3 minutes to cool a bit, then delicately detach them from the sheet.
- Leave to cool on a wire-rack.

348. Vanilla Sugar Cookies Recipe

Serving: 12 | Prep: | Cook: 8mins |Ready in:

Ingredients

- 2 cups all purpose flour
- 1/2 tsp baking powder
- 1/4 tsp salt
- 4 oz unsalted butter, room temperature
- 1 cup sugar
- 1 large egg
- 1/2 tsp vanilla

Direction

- Sift dry ingredients together.
- Cream butter and sugar.
- Beat in eggs, one at a time.
- Add vanilla.
- Add flour mixture at low speed.

- Knead dough several times; wrap in plastic and chill until firm enough to roll.
- Roll and cut as desired.
- Bake, on parchment, at 350F for 8-10 minutes.

349. Vanilla Wafer Cookies Recipe

Serving: 20 | Prep: | Cook: 12mins |Ready in:

Ingredients

- 1/2 cup butter (no substitutes) softened
- 1 cup sugar
- 1 egg
- 1 tablespoon vanilla extract
- 1 1/3 cups all purpose flour
- 3/4 teaspoon baking powder
- 1/4 teaspoon salt

Direction

- In a mixing bowl, cream butter and sugar; beat in eggs and vanilla.
- Combine dry ingredients; add to creamed mixture and mix well.
- Drop by teaspoons 2 inches apart onto ungreased baking sheets.
- Bake at 350 degrees for 12 to 15 minutes or until edges are golden brown.
- Remove to a wire rack to cool.
- Yield: about 3-1/2 dozens

350. Walnut Butterscotch Cookies Recipe

Serving: 12 | Prep: | Cook: 30mins |Ready in:

Ingredients

- 1 egg
- 1 cup brown sugar

- 1/3 cup salad oil
- 3/4 cup flour
- 1 teaspoon baking powder
- 1/2 teaspoon salt
- 1 teaspoon vanilla
- 3/4 cup broken nuts

Direction

- Sift dry ingredients.
- Beat egg then add sugar and oil then vanilla.
- Add sifted dry ingredients and nuts then put into greased square baking pan.
- Bake at 350 for 30 minutes then cut into squares when cooled.

351.   White Chocolate Cookies Recipe

Serving: 12 | Prep: | Cook: 25mins | Ready in:

Ingredients

- 200g plain flour
- 150g caster sugar
- 140g butter
- 1 egg
- 1 tsp baking powder
- 1/2 tsp vanilla extract
- 150g white chocolate chips/chunks
- 100g chopped glace cherries (optional)

Direction

- Preheat the oven to 180c. Lightly grease two baking sheets.
- Cream together the butter and sugar until pale and fluffy.
- Beat in the egg and vanilla.
- Sieve the flour, and baking powder into the mixture and add the chocolate chips and/or glace cherries and mix together
- Split the mixture into 12 balls and place on baking trays, ensure there is a lot of space between each cookie as they spread out a lot.

- Cook for 12-15 minutes until golden brown.

352.   Windmill Cookies Recipe

Serving: 10 | Prep: | Cook: 10mins | Ready in:

Ingredients

- 1 cup dates chopped
- 1/2 cup granulated sugar
- 1/2 cup water
- 2 tablespoons lemon juice
- 1/2 teaspoon salt
- Dough:
- 2 cups brown sugar firmly packed
- 1 cup shortening melted
- 2 eggs beaten
- 1 cup sour milk
- 2 cups whole wheat flour
- 2-1/2 cups flour
- 1/2 teaspoon baking soda
- 1 teaspoon ground cinnamon

Direction

- Simmer dates, sugar and water for 5 minutes then stir in lemon juice and salt.
- Set aside then preheat oven to 375 and grease a cookie sheet.
- Mix sugar and shortening then blend in eggs and milk.
- Sift together flours, baking soda and cinnamon then add to sugar mixture mixing well.
- If necessary add more flour to make dough stiff enough to roll out.
- Roll dough 1/8" thick on a floured surface and cut out cookies with a round cookie cutter.
- Place 1/2 of the cookie rounds on the cookie sheet and top each with a spoonful of filling.
- Add top cookie round which has been decorated by four small knife slits at right angles.
- Bake 10 minutes then transfer to wire rack to cool completely.

353. Yellow Cake Cookies Recipe

Serving: 8 | Prep: | Cook: 6mins | Ready in:

Ingredients

- 1 box yellow cake mix
- 3 eggs
- 1/3 cup oil
- chocolate icing (if desired)

Direction

- Preheat oven to 375.
- Combine all three ingredients.
- Pinch off dough into small balls and set about 2 inches apart on cookie sheet.
- Bake for 5 to 7 minutes or until they're golden brown around the edges.
- They're really tasty plain, but if desired, after the cookies cool, spread chocolate icing on the bottom of one cookie and put the bottom of another cookie on top to make a sandwich.

354. Your In A Jam Cookie Recipe

Serving: 24 | Prep: | Cook: 10mins | Ready in:

Ingredients

- 8-oz cream cheese
- 2 Stick oleo
- 2 Cups flour
- jam
- confectioners' sugar

Direction

- Soften the Oleo and Cream Cheese to room temperature, blend together.
- Add flour until blended thoroughly.
- Chill overnight.
- Roll out on floured surface.
- Cut in small rounds.
- Drop about 1/2 teaspoon jam in center.
- Moisten edges with water.
- Seal in a turnover shape.
- Bake on ungreased cookie sheet, at 400 degrees from anywhere between 5 to 10 minutes.
- Sprinkle or roll in confectioners' sugar.
- There are so many different, unique, fine jams to be had now days.
- Let your imagination go wild on the flavors.

355. Angel Cookies Recipe

Serving: 28 | Prep: | Cook: 10mins | Ready in:

Ingredients

- 1 boxed angel food cake mix
- 3/4 cup sugar free preserves- any flavor
- 3 tablespoons mini chocolate chips

Direction

- Mix dry cake mix with preserves until well combined.
- Stir in chocolate chips.
- Drop batter by spoonful onto greased cookie sheet.
- Bake at 325 degrees for 10 minutes.

356. Anis Seed Cookies Recipe

Serving: 2 | Prep: | Cook: 15mins | Ready in:

Ingredients

- 1 tsp.cold water
- 4 egg yokes
- 1 cup sugar
- 1 cup flour 1 tsp. anis seed

Direction

- Add cold water to egg yolks and beat until just mixed
- Add sugar. Place over hot water (not boiling) and beat until mixture thickens,
- Remove from fire and add flour and anise seed.
- Drop by spoonful on a greased cookie sheet.
- Let stand overnight in a cold oven to dry out.
- Next day remove from oven and heat oven to 300f, then bake 15-20 minutes or till cookies start to brown around the edges.

---

357.   Chewy Molasses Cookies Recipe

Serving: 30 | Prep: | Cook: 8mins | Ready in:

Ingredients

- 3/4 c butter
- 1 c sugar
- 1/4 c molasses
- 2 T honey
- 1 egg
- 2 t baking soda
- 2 1/4 c flour
- 1/4 t ground cloves
- 3/4 t ground ginger
- 1 1/2 t cinnamon

Direction

- Melt butter.
- Mix in sugar, molasses, and honey. Beat very well.
- Add egg. Beat very well. Mixture will be rather runny.
- Add baking soda, flour and spices and mix thoroughly.
- Chill dough at least 15 m.
- Preheat oven to 350 degrees.
- Shape dough into balls the size of small walnuts and roll in sugar.

- Place on greased/silpat/parchment paper lined baking sheet about 2" apart.
- Bake at 350 degrees 7-8 minutes, rotating the cookie sheet halfway through.
- Take out of the oven when they have puffed and the tops are set--do not over bake!! Cool 2-5 min on the cookie sheet, then remove to a cooling rack. If they are too hard, bake in a cooler oven, say 340, or watch them more closely. If they are too cakey, use 2 T less flour (next time, obviously).
- Store in an airtight container. The butter will keep them from sticking to each other :--)

---

358.   Chocolate Chip Cookies Recipe

Serving: 20 | Prep: | Cook: 30mins | Ready in:

Ingredients

- 1/2 cup soft butter
- 3/4 cup brown sugar
- 1 egg
- 1/2 tsp vanilla
- 1/4 tsp salt
- 1/4 tsp baking soda
- 2 tbsp corn starch
- 1 cup flour
- 1/2 cup chocolate chips

Direction

- Preheat oven to 350*
- In large bowl mix all ingredients in order shown
- Using a spoon, drop1" lumps of cookie dough on ungreased baking pan (not too close they do rise!)
- Bake for 8-10 min or until lightly brown on edges
- Let cool before removing from pan or chocolate smudges

359.   Light Peanutbutter Cookies Recipe

Serving: 2 | Prep: | Cook: 10mins | Ready in:

Ingredients

- 1 3/4 cup flour
- 3/4 tsp. baking soda
- 1/4 tsp. salt
- 1/3 cup packed light brown sugar or{diabetic Brown sugar}
- 1/3 cup Splenda sweetner or 1/3 cup sugar
- 1/4 cup butter or 1/4 cup I cant believe its not butter {original vegetable oil spread
- 2/3 cup reduce fat chunky peanut butter
- 2 egg whites
- 2 tbs. chopped peanuts

Direction

- Preheat oven 350
- Line baking sheets with foil coat with cooking spray combined
- Flour soda salt reserve
- On medium speed beat brown sugar sweetener and vegetable oil spread until creamy 1-2 minutes, beat in peanut butter and egg whites until smooth on low speed beat flour mixture until just combined
- Roll dough into 24 balls place 3 inches apart on pans using forks flatten each ball to 1/2-inch thickness press few peanuts into each center of cookie bake 9-11 minutes or till edges are set and light brown cool 5 minutes transfer from pans to racks cool completely

360.   No Bake Cookies Recipe

Serving: 2 | Prep: | Cook: 7mins | Ready in:

Ingredients

- 2 c sugar
- 1/4 c butter
- 1/2 c milk
- 1/4 c cocoa powder
- 1/2 c peanut butter
- 1 tbs vanilla
- 3 c rolled oats

Direction

- Bring first four ingredients to a full boil on med heat in a sauce pan.
- Turn off heat.
- Stir thoroughly so all ingredients are mixed and melted.
- Add the last of the ingredients.
- After combined quickly put tbsp. or your desired amount onto foil or parchment paper.
- Let cool and enjoy the cookies.

361.   No Bake Fudgey Oat Cookies Recipe

Serving: 3 | Prep: | Cook: | Ready in:

Ingredients

- 2 1/4 cup quick cooking oats
- 1 cup flake coconut
- 1/2 cup milk
- 1/4 cup butter or margirine
- 2 cups sugar
- 1/2 cup baking cocoa
- 1 tsp. vanilla
- 1/2 cup finely chopped peanuts

Direction

- In a bowl combine:
- Oats, coconut and Peanuts
- In a Saucepan:
- Combine Milk and butter
- Stir in: sugar and cocoa
- Mix well. Bring to a boil Add Oat mixture stirring constantly

- Cook for 1 minute
- Remove from heat Stir in Vanilla drop by rounded teaspoonsfuls; 1 inch apart onto waxed paper. Cool
- Makes APP. 3 dozen

362. Orange And Almond Cookies Recipe

Serving: 45 | Prep: | Cook: 45mins | Ready in:

Ingredients

- 200g butter chopped
- 1 tbls finely grated orange rind
- 1 cup (160g) icing sugar mixture
- 2 tsp orange flower water
- 2 eggs lightly beaten
- 2 cups (300g) plain flour
- 2 1/2 cups (310g) ground almonds
- 1/4 cup (40g) blanched almonds halved

Direction

- Beat butter, rind, sifted icing sugar and orange flower water in a bowl with electric mixer until light and fluffy. Add eggs gradually, beat until just combined. Transfer mixture to a large bowl. Stir in sifted flour and ground almonds, mix to a soft dough. Wrap dough in plastic and refrigerate 30 minutes.
- Roll tablespoons of mixture into balls. place about 4 cm apart on greased oven trays, flatten slightly, press halved nuts into centres bake cookies in moderate oven about 15 minutes or until lightly browned. Cool cookies on trays. Makes about 45

363. Really Easy Shortbread Recipe

Serving: 30 | Prep: | Cook: 20mins | Ready in:

Ingredients

- 1 1/2 cups of very soft butter
- 2 3/4 cups flour
- 3/4 cup of icing sugar

Direction

- Sift the icing sugar
- Cream the icing sugar and butter together until smooth
- Gradually add the flour... a little at a time... ... mixing thoroughly after each addition
- Pat the mixture into a 13 x 9 pan and prick the mixture several times with a fork
- Bake in a 350-degree oven for 20 minutes or until the edges are slightly brown.
- Let cool and cut into small squares

364. Semolina Cake Recipe

Serving: 2030 | Prep: | Cook: 22mins | Ready in:

Ingredients

- 1 can sweetened condensed milk (39g)
- 2 1/2 cups hot water
- 4 tbsp. butter
- 3/4 cup semolina
- 1 cup coconut milk (prepared)
- 1 tsp. cinnamon
- icing sugar

Direction

- Dissolve Sweetened Condensed Milk thoroughly in hot water.
- Heat butter in a medium pan and add semolina and Coconut Milk.
- Cook, stirring constantly for about 5 minutes or until semolina is lightly browned. Remove from heat.
- Gradually stir in the hot Sweetened Condensed Milk mixture into the semolina mixture and add cinnamon.

- Then stir over heat until it boils, reduce heat, then cook again, stirring for 1 minute.
- Remove from heat. Cover pan for 15 minutes.
- Grease a high-sided oven tray. Spread mixture evenly into it and stand for 10 minutes.
- Turn onto a board and cut into squares to serve.
- Dust with icing sugar or cinnamon or place some nuts on top.

365. Walnut Oat Biscuits Cookies Recipe

Serving: 15 | Prep: | Cook: 15mins | Ready in:

Ingredients

- 100g - 4 oz butter softened
- 85g - 3oz muscovado sugar
- 1 egg beaten
- 50g - 2oz porridge oats
- 50g - 2 oz walnuts, finely chopped
- 85g - 3oz plain flour
- 1/2 tsp baking powder
- cheese and strawberries to serve

Direction

- Preheat oven to 180C - gas 4
- Butter 2 baking sheets
- Beat the butter and sugar in a bowl till light and fluffy
- Stir in the oats, flour, baking powder and nuts
- Drop desert spoonfuls onto a baking sheet
- Bake for 15 min until pale golden and cool on a wire wrack

Index

Conclusion

Thank you again for downloading this book!

I hope you enjoyed reading about my book!

If you enjoyed this book, please take the time to share your thoughts and post a review on Amazon. It'd be greatly appreciated!

Write me an honest review about the book – I truly value your opinion and thoughts and I will incorporate them into my next book, which is already underway.

Thank you!

If you have any questions, **feel free to contact at:** *author@ciderrecipes.com*

Karen Hall

ciderrecipes.com

Made in the USA
Las Vegas, NV
31 January 2025